Plantæ Favershamienses. A Catalogue of the More Perfect Plants Growing Spontaneously About Faversham, in the County of Kent. With an Appendix Exhibiting a Short View of the Fossil Bodies of the Adjacent Island of Shepey. By Edward Jacob, Esq; F.S.A

Presented
by
Nottingham
July 4 1790

PLANTÆ FAVERSHAMIENSES.

A

CATALOGUE

OF THE

MORE PERFECT

PLANTS

Growing fpontaneoufly about

FAVERSHAM,

IN THE

COUNTY OF KENT.

WITH AN

APPENDIX

Exhibiting a SHORT VIEW of the

FOSSIL BODIES

OF THE ADJACENT

ISLAND OF SHEPEY.

By EDWARD JACOB, Efq; FSA.

Confider the Lillies of the Field how they grow — Matt. vii 28.

LONDON.

Printed for the AUTHOR; by J. MARCH, on Tower-Hill.

Sold by B. WHITE, at HORACE's-HEAD, FLEET-STREET;
and T. EVANS, PATER-NOSTER-ROW.

M,DCC,LXXVII.

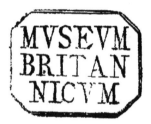

TO

Mr. JOHN WHITE,

MERCHANT OF LONDON,

IN A GRATEFUL SENSE OF HIS

LONG AND SINGULAR

FRIENDSHIP,

THIS LITTLE WORK

IS MOST RESPECTFULLY INSCRIBED

BY HIS EVER OBLIGED,

AND VERY HUMBLE SERVANT,

EDWARD JACOB.

Faverſham,
Aug. 10, 1777.

Nesço quid fascinaverit nostros ut tota mens trahatur ad peregrinas plantas, illæ vero quas pedibus conculcamus, omnino relinquuntur.

C. Linnæi Bibl. Botan p. 24.

PREFACE.

THE ensuing Collection of *PLANTS* was begun many Years since upon the Basis of the late Rev. Mr. Bateman's *Catalogue*, with whom, in the early part of Life, the Author made several *Botanical Excursions* hereabouts; and it hath gradually kept increasing ever since, as the constant Visits, in the way of his Profession, to different Parts, gave him opportunities of searching after them. It was ever intended for his own private Use and instructive Entertainment, till lately, at the recommendation of several Gentlemen well versed in Botany, it hath been revised and digested, and is now offered to the Lovers of that Science, as a means, however small, of promoting the topical Knowledge of English *Plants*; if it shall prove agreeable to their *Taste*, he will think himself amply rewarded for his Pains.

The great Promoter of its publication was the late worthy Richard Warner, *Esq*; of Wood-ford-Row, in Essex, who not only permiteed the

free

PREFACE.

free Use of his Plantæ Woodfordienses, *(without the Aid of which, and Mr.* Hudson's *excellent* Flora Anglica, *it would never have been undertaken) but also assisted the Author in the Prosecution of it, and above all, introduced him to the acquaintance of that accurate Botanist, Mr.* Alchorne, *Assay-Master of the Mint, whose kind Informations and Corrections have been of the greatest Advantage.*

The principal Inducement for the Publication was to rectify the Account given in Mr. Blackston's *Specimen Botanicum, taken from Mr.* Bateman's M.S. *Catalogue of near Two Hundred Plants growing about this Town, because many of the rare ones at this time, are not to be found in the Places therein referred to, which have of late been often diligently searched in hope of retrieving them, as they would have added much to this Work, but in vain.*

In the Course of about Seventy Years since that Catalogue was made, many Causes and Accidents may be assigned for the loss of some of the rare Plants there mentioned, yet none greater than the industrious hand of improving Husbandry. Mr. Bateman *might possibly have been mistaken in*

others,

PREFACE.

*others, and possibly too some may be overlooked by
the Author, who is not so conceited as to think he
hath discovered all the Plants growing round him.
Those Gentlemen who are fond of the Study must be
sensible, that a single Person, whose necessary attention in the different Branches of his Profession
was fully engaged, could not afford sufficient Leisure, however fervent his Inclination might be, to
search at proper Seasons every corner of a District
Five or Six Miles Diameter, when even the great
Mr.* Ray *could make considerable Additions to the
first Catalogue of his* Cambridgeshire *Plants, and
yet leave many unobserved, to be added thereto by
Dr.* Martyn, *and others.*

*In order, however, to supply his Deficiencies,
the Author hath inserted some few rare Plants
discovered at a greater distance in the Eastern
parts of the County, either by himself, or com-
municated to him by his obliging Friends, Mr.*
Alchorne, *the Rev. Mr.* Jones, *of* Pluckley,
and Mr. Boys *of* Sandwich, *for which Favours
he begs they will be pleased to accept his most
grateful Acknowledgements.*

As

PREFACE.

As he hath composed his Catalogue upon Mr. Warner's alphabetical Plan, he hopes the Preference given to Mr. Ray's Names will be pardoned by the more scientific Botanists, especially as he hath printed an Index of those of Linnæus.

The Appendix, giving a short Account of the Shepey Fossils, it is presumed will not be deemed an improper Addition, by the Lovers of Natural History, as hitherto no particular one hath been offered to their Notice, although so well deserving of it.

The Plate of the Author is the unexpected Donation of an obliging Friend.

The ABBREVIATIONS explained.

R. S. J. Raii Synopsis Stirpium Britannicarum. Ed. III. 1724.

H. F. Gul. Hudsoni Flora Anglica. 1762.

A. Annual. B. Biennial. P. Perennial. S. Shrub, or Tree.

The Month (as March, &c.) denotes the Time of the Plants flowering.

* This Mark placed before a Plant, although found wild, shews it most probably to have originated from Seed dispersed by Birds, or otherwise from Gardens.

PLANTÆ FAVERSHAMIENSES.

A

ABSINTHIUM marinum album. R. S. 188.
ARTEMISIA *maritima.* H.F. 311.
  White Sea-Wormwood.
In the Salt Marshes—very common. Auguft. P.

ABSINTHIUM vulgare. R. S 188.
  ARTEMISIA *Abfinthium.* H.F. 311.
  Common Wormwood.
In Farm-yards and on dry banks—common. Auguft. P.

* ACER majus. R S. 407.
  ACER *Pfeudo-Platanus.* H F. 378.
  The greater Maple or Sycamore Tree.
In a Hedge near Brenly *and* Hanflets Forftal — *very
uncommon.* May. S.

ACER minus. R S. 470.
  ACER *campeftre.* H. F. 379.
  The Common Maple.
In Hedges—very common. May S.

B   ACINOS.

ACINOS. R. S. 238.
THYMUS *Acinos*. H. F. 230.
Wild Bafil.
On Badgen *Downs — plentifully.* July. **A.**

ADIANTUM nigrum Officinarum. R.S. 126.
ASPLENIUM *Adiantum-nigrum*. H.F. 386.
Common black Maiden-hair.
On the hollow fandy Banks in Byfing Wood *and* Hernhill—*not common.* **P.**

AGRIFOLIUM. R. S. 466.
ILEX *Aquifolium*. H. F. 505.
The Holly Tree.
In Woods and Hedges—common. May. **S.**

AGRIMONIA. R. S. 202.
AGRIMONIA *Eupatoria*. H. F. 180.
Agrimony.
On the Sides of Fields and under Hedges — very common. June. **S.**

ALCEA vulgaris. R. S. 252.
MALVA *Alcea*. H. F. 268.
Vervain Mallow.
In Paftures at Graveney *and* Hernhill — *not common.* Auguft. **P.**

ALLIUM

ALLIUM fylveftre. R. S 369
 ALLIUM *vineale.* H. F. 121.
Crow-Garlick.
On the Wall that leads to Thorn Creek — *plentifully.*
June. P.

ALLIUM fylveftre latifolium. R. S 370.
 ALLIUM *urfinum.* H. F. 122.
Ramfons.
Amongft the Alders near Hernhill-Church — *plenti-
fully.* May. P.

ALNUS. R. S. 442.
 BETULA *Alnus.* H. F. 506.
The Common Alder.
In moift Places—very common. July. S.

ALSINE hirfuta Myofotis. R. S. 349.
 CERASTIUM *vulgatum.* H. F. 175.
Narrow-leaved Moufe-ear Chickweed.
In Fields and Meadows—common. May. A.

ALSINE hirfuta Myofotis latifolia præcocior.
 R S. 348.
 CERASTIUM *vifcofum.* H. F. 175.
The broader leaved Moufe-ear Chickweed.
On the Walls of the Abbey— common. April. A.

ALSINE major repens perennis. R. S. 347.
  CERASTIUM *aquaticum.* H. F. 177.
Great Marſh Chickweed.
In Davington *Brooks, and at* Goodneſtone — *not common.* July. P.

ALSINE marina foliis portulacæ. R.S. 351.
  ARENARIA *peploides.* H. F. 167.
Sea Chickweed
On Shellneſs *in* Shepey—*not common.* July. P.

ALSINE minor multicaulis. R. S. 349.
  ARENARIA *ſerpyllifolia.* H. F. 167.
The leaſt Chickweed.
On Roofs of old Houſes and on old Walls — common.
  May. A.

ALSINE ſpergula dicta major. R. S. 351.
  SPERGULA *arvenſis.* H. F. 177.
Corn Spurrey
On ſandy Grounds in Hern-Hill—*common.* July. A.

ALSINE ſpergulæ facie media. R. S. 351.
  ARENARIA *marina.* H. F. 169.
Sea Spurrey.
On the Paths to Holly Shore—*common.* June A.

                                      ALSINE

ALSINE foliis caryophylleis. R. S. 344.
   SAGINA *erecta*. H. F. 64.
   The leaft Stichwort.
In Nagden Marfhes—*not common.* May. A.

ALSINELLA mufcofo flore repens. R. S. 345.
   SAGINA *procumbens.* H. F 63.
   Pin Pearl-wort, Chickweed breakftone.
On old Walls about the Town—common. June. A.

ALTHÆA vulgaris. R S 252.
   ALTHÆA *officinalis.* H. F. 267.
   Marfh-Mallow.
In the Marfhes at Clapgate *and* Goodneftone—*common.* Auguft. P.

ANACAMPSEROS, vulgo Faba craffa. R.S. 269.
   SEDUM *Telephium.* H. F. 170.
   Orpine, or Live-long.
In Byfing *and* Cockfet *Woods* — *not common.* Auguft. P.

ANAGALLIS flore phœniceo. R.S. 282.
   ANAGALLIS *arvenfis.* H F. 73.
   Male Pimpernel.
In Fields and Gardens—common. May—Auguft. A.

ANAGALLIS lutea. R. S. 282.
   LYSIMACHIA *nemorum.* H. F. 73.
   Yellow Pimpernel.
In Jud's Wood, Ofpringe—*uncommon.* June. P.

ANBLATUM Cordi five Aphyllon. R. S.*288.
LATHRÆA *Squamaria.* H.F. 233.
Toothwort.

Under Hedges near Mr. Jenning's *Houfe in* Pluckley
—very uncommon. April. P.

ANEMONE nemorum. R S. 259.
ANEMONE *nemorofa.* H. F. 208.
Wood Anemony.

In Woods and Hedges—very common. April. P.

ANGELICA fylveftris R. S. 208.
ANGELICA *fylveftris.* H F. 103.
Wild Angelica.

Near Stone-Bridge, *and in* Byfing Wood — *not*
common. July P.

• ANGELICA fylveftris minor feu erratica. R.S.208.
ÆGOPODIUM *Podagraria.* H. F. 111.
Herb Gerard, Gout-weed, or Afh-weed.

In Gardens and under Hedges, near Boughton Church
—not common. May. P.

ANONIS maritima procumbens. R. S. 332.
ONONIS *repens.* H. F. 273.
Creeping Reft-harrow.

On the Sand Downs near Deal—*uncommon.* July. P

ANONIS

ANONIS ſpinoſa flore purpureo. R. S. 332.
ONONIS *ſpinoſa.* H. F. 273.
Reſt-harrow, Cammock, Petty Whin.
In the Marſhes at Clapgate—*common.* July. P.

ANONIS non ſpinoſa. R. S. 332.
ONONIS *arvenſis.* H. F. 273.
Corn Reſt-harrow, or Cammock.
In Corn Fields at Preſton *and* Oſpringe—*common.*
July. P.

ANTIRRHINUM majus. R. S. omittitur.
ANTIRRIHINUM *majus.* H. F. 239.
The greater Snap-Dragon.
On old Walls about the Town—common. June to
September. P.

APARINE. R. S. 225.
GALIUM *Aparine* H F. 57.
Cleavers, or Gooſe-graſs.
Under Hedges—very common. Auguſt. A.

APARINE paluſtris minor Pariſienſis. R. S. 225.
GALIUM *uliginoſum.* H. F. 56.
Marſh Gooſe-graſs.
At the Bottom of Jud's Wood *in* Oſpringe — *un-
common.* Auguſt. P.

APIUM

APIUM paluftre et officinarum. R. S. 214.
  APIUM *graveolens*. · H. F. 111.
  Smallage.
'*About the* Sluice Bridge *and the* Keys—*very common.*
  Auguft. B.

AQUILEGIA flore fimplici. R. S. 273.
  AQUILEGIA *vulgaris.* H. F. 207.
  Common Columbines.
In Badgen Wood, *and beyond* Whitehill, Ofpringe
  —*not common.* June. P.

ARTEMISIA vulgaris. R. S. 190.
  ARTEMISIA *vulgaris.* H. F. 312.
  Mugwort.
Under Hedges and on the Sides of Fields—very common.
  Auguft. P.

ARUM. R. S. 266.
  ARUM *maculatum.* H. F 342.
  Wake-Robin, Cuckow-Pint, Lords and Ladies.
In fhady Places and under Hedges — very common.
  May. P.

ASPERULA. R. S. 224.
  ASPERULA *odorata.* H. F. 55.
  Woodroof.
In Ofpringe Woods—*plentifully.* May. P.

ASPLE-

ASPLENIUM. R. S. 118.

ASPLENIUM *Ceterach*. H. F. 385.

Spleen-wort, Milt-waft.

On Lenham *Church Wall* — *lately loft on the Walls of our* Abbey. P.

ASTER maritimus cæruleus. R. S. 175.

ASTER *Tripolium*. H. F. 319.

Sea Star-wort.

In the Salt Marſhes—plentifully. Auguft. P.

ASTER arvenſis cæruleus acris. R. S. 175.

ERIGERON *acre*. H. F. 314.

Blue flowered Flea-bane.

On old Walls and on dry Banks—common. Auguft. P.

ASTER maritimus flavus, Crithmum chryfanthe-
mum dictus. R. S. 174.

INULA *crithmoides*. H. F. 320.

Golden Sampire.

In the Marſhes of Shepey—*uncommon.* Auguft. P.

ASTRAGALUS luteus. R. S. 326.

ASTRAGALUS *glycyphyllos*. H. F. 281.

Wild Liquorice, or Liquorice Vetch.

Under Hedges in Peaſedown, *near* Whitehill, Oſpringe
—*uncommon.* July. P.

ATRIPLEX

ATRIPLEX anguftifolia maritima dentata.
 R. S. 152.
 ATRIPLEX *ferrata.* H. F. 377.
 Narrow leaved Orache.
Near Sheernefs *in* Shepey—*uncommon.* Auguft. A.

ATRIPLEX anguftiffimo et longiffimo folio.
 R. S. 153.
 ATRIPLEX *litoralis.* H. F. 378.
 Grafs-leaved Orache.
Near Ramfgate Pier *in* Thanet —— *uncommon.*
 Auguft. A.

ATRIPLEX maritima. R. S. 152.
 ATRIPLEX *laciniata.* H. F. 376.
 Jagged Sea Orache.
Near Sheernefs *in* Shepey—*uncommon.* Auguft. A.

ATRIPLEX fylveftris anguftifolia. R. S. 151.
 ATRIPLEX *patula.* H. F. 377.
 Narrow leaved wild Orache.
In Gardens and on Dunghills—common. Auguft. A.

ATRIPLEX fylveftris folio haftato feu deltoide.
 R. S 151.
 ATRIPLEX *haftata.* H. F. 377.
 Wild Orache with a fpear pointed Leaf.
In Gardens and wafte Places — common. September. A.

ATRIPLEX

ATRIPLEX maritima ſcopariæ folio. R. S. 153.
   ATRIPLEX *litoralis.* H. F. 378. β
Graſs-leaved Orache.
Near Margate Pier *in* Thanet —— *uncommon.*
   Auguſt. A.

ATRIPLEX maritima fruticoſa. R. S. 153.
   ATRIPLEX *portulacoides.* H. F. 376.
Sea Purſlane.
Near Harty Ferry—*plentifully.* Auguſt. P.

ATRIPLEX maritima perennis folio deltoide ſeu
   triangulari. R. S. 152.
   ATRIPLEX *haſtata.* H. F. 377. β
Wild Sea Orache.
In the Brent *Marſhes—common.* Auguſt. A.

B.

BACCHARIS, monſpelienſium. R. S. 179.
   CONYZA *ſquarroſa.* H F. 314.
Plowman's Spikenard.
On Beacon Hill *and dry Banks — not uncommon.*
   Auguſt. B.

BALLOTE. R. S. 244.
   BALLOTA *nigra.* H. F. 227.
Stinking Horehound
Under Hedges—very common. Auguſt. A.

BELLA-

BELLADONNA. R. S. 265.
   ATROPA *Belladonna.* H. F. 79.
Deadly Night-fhade, or Dwale.
Amongft the Bufhes under Prefton-Houfe *Wall —
   very uncommon.* June and July. P.

BELLIS fylveftris minor. R. S. 184.
   BELLIS *perennis.* H. F. 320.
Common Daify.
In Meadows — very common. From March to Oc-
   tober. P.

BERBERIS dumetorum. R. S. 465.
   BERBERIS *vulgaris.* H F.
The Berberry-bufh, or Pipperidge-bufh.
In a Hedge beyond Queen Court, Ofpringe —— *un-
   common.* May. S.

BETONICA. R. S. 238.
   BETONICA *Officinalis.* H F. 220.
Wood Betony.
In Woods and under Hedges—common. July P.

BETA fylveftris maritima. R. S 38.
   BETA *vulgaris* H. F. 93.
Sea Beet
On the Sea Walls at Ham *and* Graveney—*uncommon.*
   Auguft. B.

                          BETULA.

BETULA. R. S. 443.
  BETULA *alba.* H. F. 354.
  The Birch Tree.
In Woods——common. April. S.

BIFOLIUM majus, feu Ophrys major quibuf-
    dam R. S. 385.
  OPHRYS *ovata.* H. F. 338.
  Common Twayblade.
In Cockfet *and* Jud's Woods—*common.* June. P.

BLITUM Atriplex fylveftris dictum. R. S. 154.
  CHENOPODIUM album. H. F. 91.
  Common wild Orache.
In uncultivated Places, and on Rubbifh——common.
    Auguft. A.

BLITUM fœtidum Vulvaria dictum. R S. 156.
  CHENOPODIUM Vulvaria. H. F. 92.
  Stinking Orache.
Under Walls about the Town—uncommon. Auguft. A.

BLITUM Ficus folio R S. 155.
  CHENOPODIUM *ferotinum.* H. F. 91.
  Late flowering or Fig-leaved Blite.
In Gardens and on Rubbifh——common. A.

C   BLITUM.

BLITUM Kali minus album dictum. R. S. 156.
 CHENOPODIUM *maritimum*. H. F. 92.
Sea Blite, or white Glafs-wort.
In the Salt Marſhes—common. Auguſt. A.

BLITUM perenne Bonus Henricus dictum.
   R S. 156.
 CHENOPODIUM *Bonus Henricus*. H.F. 89.
Common Englifh Mercury, or All-good.
By Way-ſides in Oſpringe—*not uncommon* July. P.

BLITUM Pes anſerinus dictum. R. S. 154.
 CHENOPODIUM *murale*. H. F. 90.
Common Goofe-foot, or Sow-bane.
In Gardens and on Rubbiſh —— not uncommon.
   Auguſt. A.

BLITUM Pes anſerinus dictum acutioie folio.
   R. S. 154.
 CHENOPODIUM rubrum. H. F 90.
Sharp-leaved Goofe-foot, or Sow-bane.
On Dunghills and Rubbiſh—common. Auguſt. A.

BLITUM rubrum minus. R. S. 157.
 AMARANTUS *Blitum*. H. F. 356.
The leaft Blite,
On Rubbiſh and in Gardens—common. Auguſt. A.

                                    BORRAGO

BORRAGO hortenfis. R. S. 228.
  BORRAGO *officinalis.* H. F. 68.
  Borrage.
On old Walls, and by Road-fides near the Town—
  not common. June. P.

BORRAGO fempervirens. R. S 227.
  ANCHUSA *fempervirens.* H. F. 66.
  Evergreen Alkanet.
On Rubbifh near Prefton Church Yard — *very un-*
  common. June. P.

BRASSICA maritima arborea five procerior ra-
  mofa. R. S. 293.
  BRASSICA *oleracea.* H. F 253.
  Sea Cabbage.
On the Cliffs between Deal *and* Dover — *plentifully.*
  April. B.

BRYONIA alba. R. S. 261.
  BRYONIA *alba.* H. F. 373.
  White Briony.
In Hedges — common. May. P.

BUGLOSSA fylveftris minor. R. S. 227.
  LYCOPSIS *arvenfis.* H. F. 69.
  Small wild Buglofs.
In Corn-fields near Prefton Church —— *uncommon.*
  May. A.   BUGLOS-

BUGLOSSUM arvenſe annuum. Lithoſpermi folio. R. S. 227.

LITHOSPERMUM *arvenſe*. H. F. 66.

Baſtard Alkanet.

In Corn-fields in Preſton *and* Hernhill —— *common* July. A.

BUGULA R. S. 245.

AJUGA *reptans*. H. F. 219.

Bugle.

In Byſing Wood — *common*. May. P.

BULBOCASTANUM R. S. 209.

BUNIUM *Bulbocaſtanum*. H. F. 105.

Earth-nut, or Hog-nut.

In Byſing Wood *and* Hernhill—*common*. June. P.

BUPLEURUM minimum R. S. 221.

BUPLEURUM *tenuiſſimum*. H. F 97.

The leaſt Hare's-ear.

Near Sheerneſs *in* Shepey—*uncommon*. Auguſt. A.

BUPLEURUM perfoliatum rotundifolium annuum. R. S. 221

BUPLEURUM *rotundifolium* H. F. 97.

Thorow-wax.

In Corn-fields near Brogdale *in* Oſpringe—*uncommon*. July. A.

BUTO-

BURSA Paftoris. R. S. 306.

THLASPI *Burfa Paftoris.* H. F. 247.
Shepherd's Purfe.

In Hop Grounds, and by Road-fides —— *very common.*
May *to* September. A.

BUTOMUS. R. S. 273.

BUTOMUS *umbellatus.* H. F. 152.
The flowering Rufh, or Water Gladiole.

In Dykes near Pluckley—*uncommon.* June. P.

* BUXUS. R. S. 445.

BUXUS *fempervirens.* H. F. 355.
The Box Tree.

A few large Trees near Houfes in Sheldwich —— *very*
uncommon. S.

C.

CAKILE quibufdam, aliis Eruca marina et Rhaphanus marinus. R. S. 307.

BUNIAS *Cakile.*
Sea Rocket.

Near Sheernefs *in* Shepey, *and* Cliff's End *in*
Thanet — *uncommon.* June. A.

CALAMINTHA humilior folio rotundiore.
R. S. 243.

GLECHOMA *hederacea.* H. F. 244.
Ground Ivy. Alehoof.

In fhady Places, and under Hedges — *very common.*
May. P.   CALA-

CALÀMINTHA vulgaris. R. S. 243.
MELISSA *Calamintha*. H. F. 230.
Common Calamint.
By the Sides of Roads, and under Hedges — common.
Auguſt. P.

CAMPANULA rotundifolia. R. S. 277.
CAMPANULA *rotundifolia*. H. F. 80.
The leſſer round leaved Bell Flower.
By Way-ſides in Oſpringe *and* Boughton—*not common.*
Auguſt. P.

CAMPANULA vulgatior foliis urticæ. R.S. 276.
CAMPANULA *Trachelium*. H. F. 81.
Canterbury Bells, or Great Throat-wort.
In Woods and Hedges — very common.—With a white
Flower in Hernhill *— very uncommon.* July. P.

CAPRIFOLIUM germanicum. R. S. 458.
LONICERA *Periclymenum*. H. F. 80.
Common Honey-ſuckle, or Woodbine.
In Woods and Hedges —— very common. April to
Auguſt. S.

CARDAMINE. R. S. 299.
CARDAMINE *pratenſis*. H. F. 256.
Common Ladies Smock, or Cuckow-flower.
In moiſt Meadows—very common. April. P.

CARDI-

CARDAMINE parviflora. H. F. 257.
Small flowered Ladies Smock.
In Meadows near Pluckley—*uncommon.* April. A.

CARDIACA. R. S. 239.
LEONURUS *Cardiaca.* H. F. 228.
Mother-wort.
Near Cockfet, *in* Ofpringe —— *very uncommon.*
July. B.

CARDUUS acaulos minore purpureo flore.
R S. 195.
CARDUUS *acaulos.* H. F. 308.
Dwarf Carline Thiftle.
Upon Beacon Hill—*not uncommon.* July. P.

CARDUUS caule crifpo. R. S. 194.
CARDUUS *crifpus.* H. F. 306.
Thiftle upon Thiftle.
By the Road fides, and on dry Banks in Ofpringe —
common. June. A.

CARDUUS lanceolatus. R. S. 195.
CARDUUS *lanceolatus.* H. F. 305.
Spear-Thiftle
In uncultivated Ground, and under Hedges —common.
July. B.

CARDUUS Mariæ. R. S. 195.
CARDUUS *marianus*. H. F. 307.
Milk Thiftle, or Lady's Thiftle.
By the Way-fide at Davington, *and by the Sea Walls beyond* Nagden—*not uncommon.* July. A.

CARDUUS Mariæ hirfutus -non maculatus.
R. S. 194.
CARDUUS marianus. H. F. 307. β.
Ladies Thiftle without Spots.
In Graveney *Marfhes — uncommon.* July. A.

CARDUUS nutans. R. S. 193.
CARDUUS *nutans.* H. F. 306.
Mufk Thiftle.
On Badgen Downs — *plentifully.* July. B.

CARDUUS paluftris. R. S. 194.
CARDUUS *paluftris.* H F. 306.
Marfh Thiftle.
In the Marfhes — common. July. B.

CARDUUS fpinofiffimus capitulis minoribus.
R. S. 194.
CARDUUS *acanthoides* H. F. 306.
Welted Thiftle with fmall Flowers.
Upon Graveney *Marfh Sea Wall—common.* July. A.

CAR-

CARDUUS ftellatus. R. S. 176.
  CENTAUREA *Calcitrapa.* H. F. 326.
  Star Thiftle.
In Graveney *Marfhes — common.* July. A.

CARDUUS tomentofus Acanthium di&us vul-
    garis. R. S. 196.
  ONOPORDUM *Acanthium.* H. F. 308.
  Cotton Thiftle.
In uncultivated Places, and by the Road-fide—common.
    July. B.

CARDUUS vulgatiffimus viarum. R. S. 194.
  SERRATULA *arvenfis.* H. F. 305.
  Common Way-Thiftle, or Creeping Thiftle.
In Fields and Byways — very common. July. P.

CARLINA fylveftris quibufdam, aliis Atra&ilis.
    R. S 175.
  CARLINA vulgaris. H. F. 309.
  The common wild Carline Thiftle.
In dry Fields and Paftures — common. June. B.

CARYOPHYLLATA. R. S. 253.
  GEUM *urbanum.* H. F. 198.
  Herb Bennet, or Common Avens.
In Woods, and under Hedges—common. July. P.

CARY-

CARYOPHYLLATA montana purpurea. R. S. 253.

GEUM *rivale*. H. F. 198.

Water Avens

In a Wood near Barber's Mill *in* Hothfield — *very uncommon*. July. P.

CARYOPHYLLUS holosteus arvensis glaber flore majore. R. S. 346.

STELLARIA *Holostea*. H. F. 166.

The greater Stich-wort

Under Hedges, and on the Sides of Fields —— *very common*. April. P.

CARYOPHYLLUS holosteus arvensis glaber flore minore. R. S. 346.

STELLARIA *graminea*. H. F. 166.

The lesser Stich-wort.

Under Hedges, chiefly on a dry Soil—common. July. P.

CARYOPHYLLUS holosteus arvensis medius. R. S. 347.

STELLARIA *graminea*. H. F. 166. β.

The middle Stich-wort.

Upon Beacon Hill — *not uncommon*. July. P.

CARYOPHYLLUS latifolius barbatus minor annuus flore minore. R. S. 337.

DIANTHUS *Armeria*. H. F. 161.

Deptford Pink.

On Beacon Hill, *and dry Pastures in* Ospringe — *not uncommon*. July. A.   CAS-

CASTANEA. R. S. 440.

FAGUS *Caſtanea.* H. F. 359.

The Cheſnut Tree.

a Byſing *and other* Woods—*not uncommon.* May. S.

CATANANCE leguminoſa quorundam. R. S. 325.

LATHYRUS *Niſſolia.* H. F. 275.

Crimſon Graſs-Vetch.

On Beacon Hill —— *not uncommon.* June. A.

CAUCALIS minor floſculis rubentibus. R. S. 219.

CAUCALIS *Anthriſcus.* H. F. 99.

Hedge Parſley.

In buſhy Grounds, and on Ham Wall—*not uncommon.* July. B.

CAUCALIS ſegetum minor, Anthriſco hiſpido ſimilis. R. S 220.

CAUCALIS *arvenſis.* H. F. 98.

Small Corn Parſley.

In Fields, and amongſt Corn—common. Auguſt. A.

CENTAURIUM luteum perfoliatum. R. S. 287.

BLACKSTONIA *perfoliata.* H. F. 146.

Yellow Centory.

In dry chalky Fields — *common.* July. A.

CEN-

CENTAURIUM minus. R. S. 286.

   GENTIANA *Centaurium.* H. F. 88.

   Leſſer Centory.

In dry Paſtures—very common. July to October. A.
With a white Flower, near Minſter *in* Shepey —
   but uncommon.

CERASUS ſylveſtris fructu rubro. R. S. 463.

   PRUNUS *Avium.* H. F. 187.

   Common wild Cherry.

In Woods —— common. April. S.

CERASTIUM hirſutum minus parvo flore.
   R. S. 348.

   CERASTIUM *ſemi-decandrium.* H. F. 175.

   The leaſt Mouſe-ear Chickweed

On Walls and dry Soils — common. April. A.

CEREFOLIUM ſylveſtre. R. S. 207.

   CHÆROPHYLLUM *temulum.* H. F. 108.

   Wild Chervil.

Under Hedges — very common. July. A.

CHAMÆMELUM *fœtidum.* R. S. 185.

   ANTHEMIS *Cotula.* H. F. 223.

   Stinking Mayweed.

In Corn Fields —— too common. June. A.

CHA-

CHAMÆMELUM inodorum. R. S. 185.
MATRICARIA *inodora*. H.F. 322.
Field Feverfew.
On the fides of paths in Corn-fields —— *common.*
Auguft. A.

CHAMÆMELUM odoratiffimum repens flore
fimplici. R. S. 185.
ANTHEMIS *nobilis*. H. F. 323.
Sweet-fcented Camomile.
On Charing Heath—*uncommon.* Auguft. P.

CHAMÆMELUM vulgare. R. S 184.
MATRICARIA *Chamomilla.* H.F. 322.
Córn Feverfew.
In cultivated Fields amongft Corn—common. June. A.

CHELIDONIUM minus. R S 246.
FICARIA *verna.* H. F 214.
Pilewort, or leffer Celandine.
In Meadows — very common. April. P.

CHENOPODIUM Betæ folio. R. S. 157.
CHENOPODIUM *polyfpermum.* H F. 92.
Upright round leaved Blite, or Allfeed.
In the Conduit Row—*not uncommon.* Auguft. A.

D   CHENO-

CHENOPODIUM erectum foliis triangularibus dentatis, fpicis e foliorum alıs plurimıs longis erectis tenuibus. R. S. 155.
CHENOPODIUM *urbıcum*. H. F. 89.
Upright Blite.
In the Conduit Row, *and ın Ditches—common.* September. A.

CHENOPODIUM Stramonii folıo. R. S. 154.
CHENOPODIUM *hybrıdum*. H. F. 90.
Maple-leaved Blite.
On Dunghills—not common. Auguft. A.

CHRYSANTHEMUM fegetum. R. S. 182.
CHRYSANTHEMUM *fegetum*. H. F. 321.
Corn Marıgold.
In Corn-fields —— common. July. A.

CICHOREUM fylveftre. R. S. 172.
CICHOREUM *Intybus*. H. F. 303.
Wıld Succory.
In uncultivated Places, and by Sıdes of Fields——very common. Auguft. P.

CICUTA. R. S. 215.
CONIUM maculatum. H. F. 100.
Hemlock.
In fhady Places near the Town—*common.* July. A.

CICUTARIA tenuifolia. R. S. 215.
ÆTHUSA *Cynapium.* H. F. 107.
The leſſer Hémlock, or Fools Parſley.
In Gatefield, *and in Gardens — not uncommon.* September. A.

CICUTARIA vulgaris. R. S. 207.
CHÆROPHYLLUM *ſylveſtre.* H. F. 108.
Wild Cicely, or Cow-weed.
Under Hedges, and in Fields — common. June. A.

CIRCÆA lutetiana. R. S. 289.
CIRCÆA *lutetiana.* H. F. 9.
Enchanters Night-ſhade.
In Byſing Wood — *common.* July. P.

CLEMATIS daphnoides major. R. S. 268.
VINCA *major.* H. F. 77.
The greater Periwinkle.
In Hedges, near Houſes at Ore *and* Sindal *Farm — uncommon.* April. P.

CLEMATIS latifolia ſeu Atragene quibuſdam. R. S. 258.
CLEMATIS *Vitalba.* H. F. 217.
Great Wild Climber, or Traveller's Joy.
In Hedges —— very common. July. P.

D 2　　　　　CLINO-

CLINOPODIUM Origano fimile. R. S. 239.

CLINOPODIUM *vulgare.* H. F. 228.

. Great wild Bafil

In Hedges — *very common.* July. P.

COCHLEARIA folio finuato. R. S. 303.

COCHLEARIA *anglica.* H. F. 248.

Sea Scurvy-grafs.

On the Sea Walls near Thorn—*common.* May. B.

CONVOLVULUS major. R. S. 275.

CONVOLVULUS *fepium.* H. F. 74.

Great Bindweed.

Under Hedges—very common. With a reddifh purple
Flower, in the Brent *Hedge; but very uncommon.*
Auguft. P.

CONVOLVULUS maritimus Soldanella dictus.
R. S 276.

CONVOLVULUS *Soldanella.* H. F. 75.

Sea Bindweed

On the Sand Downs near Sandwich — *not common.*
July P.

CONVOLVULUS minor vulgaris. R. S. 275.

. CONVOLVULUS *arvenfis.* H. F. 74.

Small Bindweed.

In Fields, and by Road-fides—very common. July. P.

CONIZA

CONYZA media. R. S. 174.
  INULA *dyfenterica.* H. F. 320.
  Middle Fleabane.
About the Abbey Pond — *common.* Auguft. P.

CONYZA minor. R. S. 174.
  INULA *Pulicaria.* H. F. 320.
  Small Fleabane.
About the Conduit-row, *and at* Downe's-forftal *in*
  Hernhill — *not uncommon.* September. A.

CORNUS fæmina. R. S. 460.
  CORNUS *fanguinea.* H. F. 58.
  The female Cornel, Dog-berry Tree, or
  Prick-wood.
In Hedges —— *common.* June. S.

CORYLUS fylveftris. R. S. 439.
  CORYLUS *Avellana.* H. F. 360.
  The Hazle-nut Tree.
In Woods and Hedges —*very common.* March. S.

COTYLEDON vera radice tuberofa. R. S. 271.
  COTYLEDON *Umbilicus Veneris.* H. F. 169.
  Navel-wort, Kidney-wort, or Wall Penny-wort.
On Tenterden *Church, and in a Stone Pit at*
  Boughton Monchelfea—*very uncommon.* June. P.

CRACCA.

CRACCA. R. S. 322.
  VICIA *Cracca.* H. F. 277.
  Tufted Vetch.
In the Hedges of the Beacon *Farm* —— *uncommon.*
  July. A.

CRACCA minor. R S. 322.
  ERVUM *hirfutum.* H. F. 280.
  Small wild Tare, Tine-Tare, or hairy Tare.
In Rickefy-lane *Hedge,* Selling —— *not uncommon.*
  July. A.

CRACCA minor filiquis fingularibus flofculis
    cærulefcentibus. R. S. 322.
  ERVUM *tetrafpermum.* H. F.
  Tine-Tare with fmooth Pods, or fmooth Tare.
In Fields and under Hedges—common. June. A.

CRITHMUM marinum. R. S. 217.
  CRITHMUM *maritimum.* H. F. 101.
  Sampire.
On the Cliffs between St. Margaret's *and* Dover ——
    plentifully Auguft. P.

CRUCIATA. R S. 223.
  VALANTIA *Cruciata.* H. F. 375.
  Crofs-wort, or Mug-weed
In Hedges in Prefton *and* Ofpringe—*not uncommon.*
  June. F.

CUSCUTA

CUSCUTA major. R. S. 281.
  CUSCUTA *europæa*. H. F. 89.
  Dodder, Hell-weed, Devil's-guts.
Upon leguminous Plants —— *common.* July. A.

CYANUS. R. S. 198.
  CENTAUREA *Cyanus*. H F. 325.
  Blue Bottles, or Corn Bottles.
In Corn-fields —— *very common.* July. A.

CYNOGLOSSUM. R. S. 226.
  CYNOGLOSSUM *officinale*. H. F. 67. β.
  Great Hound's Tongue.
By the Road Sides near Boughton Chalk Pits —— *not*
  common. June. P.

CYNOGLOSSUM folio virenti. R. S. 226.
  CYNOGLOSSUM *officinale* H. F. 67. β.
  The lesser green leaved Hound's Tongue.
Near Sandwich —— *not common.* June. P.

D.

DAMASONIUM stellatum Dalechampii.
  R. S 272.
  ALISMA *Damasonium*. H. F. 138.
  Star-headed Water Plantain.
In a Field-pond of Mr Jacob's *Farm, at* East Church
  in Shepey—*very uncommon.* June to August. P.

DAU-

DAUCUS vulgaris. R. S. 218.
DAUCUS *Carota.* H F. 99.
Wild Carrot, or Bird's Neft.
In Paftures, and by Way-fides—very common. July. B.

* DELPHINIUM fegetum flore caruleo.
  R. S. 273.
  DELPHINIUM *Confolida.* H. F. 207.
  Wild Larkfpur.
In King's Field, *amougft Corn —— very uncommon.*
June. A.

DENS-LEONIS. R. S. 170.
  LEONTODON *Taraxacum.* H. F. 297.
  Dandelion.
In Meadows and Paftures—very common. May. P.

DENS-LEONIS hirfutus, Hieracium dictus.
  R. S. 127.
  LEONTODON *hifpidum.* H. F. 297.
  Rough Dandelion, or Dandelion Hawk-weed.
In Meadows and Paftures — common. June. P.

DIGITALIS purpurea R. S. * 283.
  DIGITALIS *purpurea.* H. F 240.
  Purple Fox Glove.
In Woods and Hedges — common. Ju'y. B.

       DIPSACUS

DIPSACUS minor feu Virga paftoris. R. S. 192.
   DIPSACUS *pilofus*. H. F. 49.
Small wild Teafel, or Shepherd's Rod.
In the Road Hedge leading from Plomford *to* Badgen
   Downs — *uncommon.* July or Auguft. B.

DIPSACUS *fylveftris* feu Labrum Veneris.
   R. S. 192.
   DIPSACUS *fylveftris*. H. F. 49.
Wild Teafel.
In uncultivated Places, and under Hedges —— *very
   common.* July. B.

E.

ECHIUM alterum five Lycopfis anglica. R. S. 228.
   ECHIUM *anglicum*. H. F. 70.
Englifh Viper's Buglofs.
By Way fides near Whitehill *in* Ofpringe — *not un-
   common.* Auguft. P.

ECHIUM vulgare. R. S. 218.
   ECHIUM *vulgare*. H. F. 69.
Viper's Buglofs.
On barren Ground, and upon old Walls — *very common.*
   July. P.

EQUISETUM arvenfe longioribus fetis. R. S.
   130.
   EQUISETUM *arvenfe*. H. F. 380.
Corn Horfe-tail.
In moift Fields amongft Corn — *common.* March. P.

EQUISETUM majus. R. S. 130.
  EQUISETUM *fluviatile.* H. F. 381.
  River Horfe-tail.
In the River about the Powder Mills —— *common.*
    May. P.

EQUISETUM paluftre. R. S. 131.
  EQUISETUM *paluftre.* H. F. 380.
  The lefler Marfh Horfe-tail.
In the Corn Fields near Nagden —— *not uncommon.*
    June. P.

EQUISETUM fylvaticum. R. S. 130.
  EQUISETUM *fylvaticum.* H. F. 380.
  Wood Horfe-tail.
In the fwampy Ground near Ore Mill — *not common.*
    May. P.

ERICA Brabantica folio Coridis hirfuto quaterno.
    R. S. 471.
  ERICA *tetralix.* H. F. 144.
  Crofs-leaved Heath.
At the Bottom of Jud's Wood — *not common.* Au-
    guft. S.

ERICA tenuifolia. R. S. 471.
  ERICA *cinerea.* H. F. 144
  Fine leaved Heath.
Upon Charing Heath — *not common.* Auguft. S.

ERICA

ERICA vulgaris. R. S. 470.
  ERICA *vulgaris*. H. F. 144.
  Common Heath, or Ling.
In Woods—very common. June to September. P.

ERUCA aquatica. R. S. 297.
  SISYMBRIUM *sylvestre*. H. F. 258.
  Water Rocket.
In Ham Ponds *near* Sandwich—*uncommon.* June. P.

ERUCA hirsuta siliqua cauli appressa. Erysimum
    vulgare. R. S. 298.
  ERYSIMUM *officinale*. H. F. 250.
  Hedge Mustard.
Under Hedges, and by Road Sides —— *very common.*
    May. A.

ERUCA lutea seu Barbarea. R. S. 297.
  ERYSIMUM *Barbarea*. H. F. 251.
  Winter Cress or Rocket.
Near the Powder Mills—*not uncommon.* May. P.

ERYNGIUM marinum. R. S. 222.
  ERYNGIUM *maritimum*. H. F. 95.
  Eryngo, or Sea Holly.
On the Shore between Graveney *and* Sea Salter ——
    uncommon. July. P.

ERYSIMUM

ERYSIMUM Sophia dictum. R. S. 298.
  SYSIMBRIUM *Sophia*. H. F. 259.
  Flix-weed.
By the Road Sides near Sittingbourn —— *uncommon*.
    June. A.

EUONYMUS vulgaris. R. S. 468.
  EUONYMUS *europæus*. H. F. 84.
  The Spindle Tree, or Prick-wood.
In Woods and Hedges —common. May. S.

EUPATORIUM Cannabinum. R. S. 179.
  EUPATORIUM *cannabium*. H. F. 310.
  Common Hemp Agrimony, or Dutch Agrimony.
About the Abbey Pond*—common*. Auguft. P.

EUPHRASIA. R. S. * 284.
  EUPHRASIA *officinalis*. H. F. 234.
  Eye-bright.
In moft upland Paftures—very common. Auguft. A.

EUPHRASIA pratenfis rubra. R. S. * 284.
  EUPHRASIA *Odontites*. H. F. 234.
  Red Eye-bright.
In the Ways and Corn Fields about Prefton——*very*
    common. Auguft. A.

                                    FAGUS.

F.

FAGUS. R. S. 439.
 FAGUS *sylvaticus*. H. F. 360.
 The Beech Tree.
In Woods —— common. May. S.

* FEGOPYRUM. R. S. 144.
  POLYGONUM *Fagopyrum.* H.F. 150.
  Buck-wheat, or Brank.
In Corn fields near Beacon Hill—*uncommon.* July. A.

FEGOPYRUM scandens sylvestre. R. S. 144.
 POLYGONUM *Convolvulus.* H.F. 149.
 Black Bind-weed.
In Corn fields and Hedges — not uncommon. June to
 September. A.

FERRUM equinum germanicum siliquis in sum-
  mitate. R S. 326.
  HIPPOCREPIS *comosa.* H. F. 281.
  Tufted Horse-shoe Vetch.
On chalky Ground in Ospringe—*common.* July. A.

FILIPENDULA. R S 259.
 SPIRÆA *Filipendula.* H. F. 190.
 Common Dropwort.
Upon Beacon Hill — *not uncommon.* July. P.

E

FILIX

FII IX Fœmina.   R. S. 124.
   PTERIS *aquilina.*   H. F. 384.
   Female Fern, or Common Brakes.
In Woods —— very common.   Auguft.   P.

FILIX mas vulgaris.   R. S. 120
   POLYPODIUM *Filix mas.*   H. F. 389.
   Common Male Fern.
On fhady Banks under Hedges — common.   P.

FILICULA faxatilis ramofa maritima noftras.
      R. S. 125.
   PTERIS *aquilina.*   H. F. 384. β.
   Small-branched Stone-Fern.
On Walls about the Town*—uncommon.*   Auguft.   P.

FŒNICULUM vulgare.   R. S. 217.
   ANETHUM *Fœniculum.*   H. F. 110.
   Common Fennel, or Finkle.
By the Road-fide as you enter the Town*—not uncom-
      mon.*   Auguft.   P.

FRAGARIA.   R. S. 254.
   FRAGARIA *vefca.*   H. F. 194.
   Strawberry.
In Woods — very common.   April.   P.

FRAGRA-

FRAGARIA sterilis   R. S. 254.
  FRAGARIA *sterilis*.   H. F. 195.
  Barren Strawberry.
On barren Lands — very common.   April.   P.

FRANGULA sive Alnus nigra baccifera.   R
     465.
  RHAMNUS *Frangula*.   H. F. 83.
  The black Berry-bearing Alder.
In Badgen Wood — *not common.*   May.   S.

FRAXINUS.   R. S.   469.
  FRAXINUS *excelsior*.   H. F. 379.
  The common Ash Tree.
In Woods and Hedges — common.   April.   S.

FUMARIA vulgaris.   R. S. 204.
  FUMARIA *officinalis*.   H. F. 270.
  Fumitory.
In Fields and Gardens — common.   May.   A.

FUMARIA alba latifolia.   R. S. 204.
  FUMARIA *claviculata*.   H. F. 270.
  Climbing Fumitory.
In moist Hedges in Davington *and* Ospringe —— *not*
     common.   August.   A.

GALE

G.

GALE frutex odoratus feptentrionalium. R.S. 443
   MYRICA *Gale*. H. F. 368.
   Sweet Willow, Goule, Dutch Myrtle.
On Willfborough Lees, *near* Afhford — *plentifully*.
   May. S.

GALEOPSIS legitima Diofcoridis. R. S. 237.
   STACHYS *fylvatica*. H. F. 227.
   Hedge Nettle.
In Woods and Hedges—very common. Auguft. A.

GALLIUM luteum. R. S. 224.
   GALLIUM *verum*. H. F. 55.
   Yellow Ladies Bedftraw, or Cheefe-renning.
On the Sides of Fields—very common. July. P.

GENISTA angulofa trifolia. R. S. 474.
   SPARTIUM *fcoparium*. H. F. 271.
   Common Broom.
In Woods and dry Fields — very common. June. P.

GENISTA minor afpalathoides. R. S. 475.
   GENISTA *anglica*. H. F. 272.
   Needle Furze, or Petty Whin.
Amongft Furze which grows on wet Land ——— not
   common. May. P.

GENISTA

GENISTA fpinofa vulgaris.　R. S. 475.
ULEX *europæus*.　H. F. 272.
Furze, Whins, or Gorfe.
On Beacon Hill—*very common.*　March to June.　P.

GENISTELLA tinctoria.　R. S. 474.
GENISTA *tinctoria*.　H. F. 272.
Dyers-weed, Green-wood.
In the Marfhes near Holly Shore —— *not common.*
July.　P.

GENTIANELLA fugax autumnalis. R.S. 275.
GENTIANA *Amarella*.　H. F 87.
Autumnal Gentian.
In dry Paftures and Ofpringe Chalk Pits —— *not
uncommon*　Auguft.　A.

GERANIUM Cicutæ folio inodorum.　R. S. 357.
GERANIUM *cicutarium*.　H F. 262
Field Crane's-bill without Scent, or Hemlock-
leaved Crane's-bill.
By Road fides, and on old Walls —— *not uncommon.*
April to June.　A.

GERANIUM columbinum.　R. S. 359.
GERANIUM *molle*　H. F. 265.
Common Dove's-foot Crane's bill
Under Hedges — very common.　June.　A.

E 3　　　　　　GERA-

GERANIUM columbinum humile flore cæruleo.
R. S. 359.
GERANIUM *pufillum.* H. F. 266.
Small flowered Dove's-foot Crane's-bill.
By Wayfides leading to Thorn —*common.* June. A.

GERANIUM columbinum majus foliis diffectis.
R. S. 359.
GERANIUM *diffectum.* H. F. 266.
Jagged leaved Dove's-foot Crane's-bill.
In dry Fields in Ofpringe — *not uncommon.* May to
July. A.

GERANIUM columbinum diffectis foliis pediculis
florum longiffimis R S. 359.
GERANIUM *columbinum.* H. F. 266.
Long-ftalked Dove's-foot Crane's-bill.
Upon Oldwives Lees — *not common.* July. A.

GERANIUM robertianum. R. S. 358.
GERANIUM *robertianum.* H. F. 264.
Herb Robert.
In Hedge·, and on Rubbifh—*very common.* June. B

GERANIUM pufillum fupinum maritimum.
R. S. 357.
CERANIUM *maritimum.* H F 263.
Sea Crane's-bill.
On the Sand Downs near Deal —— *not common.*
Avguft. P. GLAUX

GLAUX maritima. R. S. 285.
GLAUX *maritima*, H. F. 86.
Sea Milkwort, or black Saltwort.
In the Brent *Marshes — common.* July. P.

GNAPHALIUM longifolium humile ramofum
    capitulis nigris. R. S. 181.
GNAPHALIUM *uliginofum*. H. F. 313.
Black-headed, long leaved, low branched cud-
    weed
In moist Places in Hernhill —— *not uncommon.*
    Auguft. A.

GNAPHALIUM anglicum. R. S. 180.
GNAPHALIUM *fylvaticum*. H. F. 313.
Upright Cudweed.
In Judd's Wood— *common.* Auguft. B.

GNAPHALIUM minimum. R. S. 181.
FILAGO *montana*. H. F. 328.
The leaft Cudweed.
In dry fandy Meadows, and among Corn —— common.
    July. A.

GNAPHALIUM minus feu Herba impia.
    R S 180.
FILAGO *germanica*. H. F. 328.
Common Cudweed.
In dry Meadows and by Road fides—common. July. A.

GROS-

* GROSSULARIA. Miller Botan Officinal. 220.
RIBES *Uva crispa.* Lin. Syftem. Nat. *Tom.* II.
    p. 184.
The Goofeberry Bufh.
In feveral Hedges beyond White Hill, Ofpringe.
April. S.

H.

HEDERA communis major et minor. R. S. 459.
HEDERA *Helix.* H. F. 85.
Climbing, or berried Ivy, alfo barren and creeping
    Ivy.
In Woods and Hedges — very common. October. S.

HELIANTHEMUM vulgare. R. S. 341.
CISTUS *Helianthemum.* H. F. 205.
Dwarf Ciftus, or little Sunflower.
On dry chalky Banks — very common. June. P.

HELENIUM. R. S. 176.
INULA *Helenium.* H. F. 319.
Elicampane.
On the moift Ground near the Half-way Houfe to Can-
    terbury — *very uncommon.* Auguft. P.

HELLEBORUS niger hortenfis. R. S. 271.
HELLEBORUS *viridis.* H. F. 215.
Wild black Hellebore.
On the Cliff beyond Weftfield *in* Pluckley —— *un-*
    common. April. P.   HEL·

HELLEBORASTER maximus. R. S. 271.
  HELLEBORUS *fœtidus*. H. F. 215.
  Great baftard black Hellebore, Bear's-foot, or
    Setter-wort.
By the Road fide, up the Chalk-hill, *about a Mile*
  North-weft from Charing—*uncommon*. March. P.

HELLEBORINE altera atro-rubente flore.
    R. S. 383.
  SERAPIAS *latifolia*. H. F. 341. β.
  Broad-leaved baftard Hellebore, a Variety.
In Ofpringe Woods——*uncommon*. Auguft. P.

HELLEBORINE latifolia montana. R. S. 383.
  SERAPIAS *latifolia*. H. F. 341.
  Broad leaved baftard Hellebore.
In King's Wood—*uncommon*. July. P.

HELLEBORINE latifolia flore albo claufo.
    R. S. 384.
  SERAPIAS *longifolia*. H. F. 341.
  White flowered baftard Hellebore.
In Badgen *and* Jud's Woods—*uncommon*. June. P.

HERBA Paris. R. S. 264.
  PARIS *quadrifolia*. H. F. 150.
  Herb Paris, True-love, or One-berry.
In Woods near Doddington—*not common*. May. P.

                                        HES-

HESPERIS allium redolens. R. S. 293.

ERYSIMUM *Alliaria.* H. F. 251.

Jack by the Hedge, or Sauce alone

Under Hedges — very common. May. P.

HIERACIUM Echioides capitulis Cardui bene-
dicti. R. S. 166.

PICRIS *Echioides.* H. F. 294.

Ox's Tongue, or Lang de Boeuf.

In Hedges and Pastures going to Thorn Creek ——
common. July. A.

HIERACIUM fruticosum angustifolium majus.
R. S. 168.

HIERACIUM *umbellatum.* H. F. 300.

Narrow leaved bushy Hawk-weed.

In Ospringe *Chalk Pits, and by Way-sides at* Dunkirk
— uncommon. August. P.

HIERACIUM fruticosum latifolium hirsutum.
R. S. 187.

HIERACIUM *sabaudum.* H. F. 300.

Bushy Hawk-weed with broad rough Leaves.

In Hedges about Sheldwich *— not common.* July. P.

HIERACIUM longius radicatum. R. S. 165.

HYPOCHÆRIS *radicata.* H. F. 302.

Long-rooted Hawk-weed.

On Beacon Hill —— *common.* June. P.

HIER-

HIERACIUM luteum glabrum five minus hir-
  futum. R. S. 165.
  CREPIS *tectorum.* H. F. 301.
  Smooth Succory Hawk-weed.
In Fields and on old Walls — *common.* June to Sep-
  tember. A.

HIERACIUM maximum Chondrillæ folio afpe-
  rum. R. S. 166.
  CREPIS *biennis.* H. F. 301.
  Rough Succory Hawk-weed.
In Hedges near Sittingbourn—*uncommon.* Auguft. B.

HIERACIUM minus præmorfa radice. R.S. 164.
  LEONTODON *autumnale.* H. F. 297.
  Hawk-weed with bitten Roots, or yellow Devil's
  Bit.
In Corn fields in Hernhill—*common.* Auguft. P.

HORMINUM fylveftre Lavendulæ flore. R. S.
  237.
  SALVIA *verbenaca.* H. F. 9.
  Common Englifh wild Clary, or Oculus Chrifti.
In Davington *and* Ore *Church-Yards* — *not common.*
  May. P.

HOTTONIA. R. S. 285.
  HOTTONIA *paluftris* H. F. 72.
  Water Violet, or Gilliflower.
About the Decoy Ponds— *uncommon. In Dykes near*
  Deal —*common.* June. P.   HYA

HYACINTHUS anglicus. R. S. 373.

HYACINTHUS *non scriptus*. H. F. 123.

Englifh Hyacinth, or Hare-bells.

In Woods and under Hedges—very common. April. P.

HYDROCOTYLE vulgaris. R. S. 222.

HYDROCOTYLE *vulgaris*. H. F. 96.

Marfh Penny-wort, or White-rot.

In the Marfhes about Luddenham *and* Ore — *not uncommon.* May. P.

HYOSCYAMUS vulgaris. R. S. 274.

HYOSCYAMUS *niger*. H. F. 77.

Common Henbane.

By Road fides near the Town—*common.* June. P.

HYPERICUM. R. S. 342.

HYPERICUM *perforatum*. H. F. 290.

Saint John's-wort.

Under Hedges, and by Road fides —— *very common.* July. P.

HYPERICUM Androfæmum dictum. R.S. 343.

HYPERICUM *hirfutum*. H. F. 291.

Tutfan, or hairy St. John's-wort.

In hollow Lanes in Boughton—*uncommon.* July. P.

HYPE-

HYPERICUM Afcyron dictum caule quadran-
gulo. R. S. 344.
HYPERICUM *quâdrangulum*. H. F. 292.
Saint Peter's-wort.
In Davington *Brooks—not uncommon.* July. P.

HYPERICUM pulchrum Tragi. R. S. 342.
HYPERICUM *pulchrum*. H. F. 290.
Upright Saint John's-wort.
In Byfing Wood — *common.* July. P.

HYPERICUM maximum Androfæmum vulgare
dictum. R. S. 343.
HYPERICUM *Androfæmum*. H. F. 291.
Tutfan, or Park-leaves.
In a Hedge near Provender Wood —— *uncommon.*
July. P.

HYPERICUM minus fupinum. R. S. 343.
HYPERICUM *humifufum*. H. F. 290.
The least trailing Saint John's-wort.
On fandy Lands in Ore—*common.* July. P.

HYPERICUM elegantiffimum non ramofum
folio lato. R. S. 343.
HYPERICUM *montenum*. H. F. 291.
Imperforate Saint John's-wort.
In Byfing Wood — *uncommon.* July. P.

JACEA

J.

JACEA major. R. S. 198.
  CENTAUREA *Scabiofa*. H. F. 325.
  Great Knap-weed, or Matfellon.
On the fides of Paths — common. July. P.

JACEA nigra. R. S. 198.
  CENTAUREA *Jacea*. H. F. 326.
  Common Knap-weed, or Matfellon.
On the fides of Fields—very common. Auguft. P.

JACOBÆA latifolia paluftris five aquatica.
    R. S. 178.
  SENECIO *aquaticus*. H. F. 317.
  Broad-leaved Marfh or Water Ragwort.
In the Brents — *common.* Auguft. P.

JACOBÆA fenecionis folio incano perennis.
    R. S. 177.
  SENECIO *erucifolius*. H. F. 317.
  Hoary Perennial Ragwort with Groundfel Leaves.
In Byfing Wood — *not common.* July. P.

JACOBÆA vulgaris. R. S. 177.
  SENECIO *Jacobæa*. H. F. 316.
  Common Ragwort.
In Meadows and Paftures—very common. July. P.

IRIS

IRIS paluftris lutea. R. S. 374.
IRIS *Pfeudacorus.* H. F. 13.
Yellow Water Flower de luce.
In moift boggy Places — very common. June. P.

IRIS fylveftris quam Xyrim vocant. R. S. 375.
IRIS *fœtidiffima.* H. F. 13.
Stinking Gladdon.
By Sandgate Caftle *near* Folkftone—*very uncommon.*
July. P.

JUNIPERUS vulgaris baccis parvis purpureis.
R. S. 444.
JUNIPERUS *communis.* H. F. 372.
The common Juniper.
On dry chalky Commons — very common. May. S.

K.

KALI geniculatum perenne fruticofius procum-
bens. R. S. 136.
SALICORNIA *europæa.* H. F. 1. β.
Perennial Marfh Sampire, or jointed Glafs-wort.
In the Ifle *of* Shepey—*uncommon.* Auguft. P.

KALI fpinofum cochleatum. R. S. 159.
SALSOLA *Kali.* H. F. 33.
Prickly Glafs-wort.
On the Shore between Graveney *and* Seafalter — *not
common.* July. A.

KNAWEL. R. S. 159.

SCLERANTHUS *annuus.* H F. 160.

German Knot-grafs, or annual Knawel.

On barren dry fandy Soils—very common. Auguſt. A.

L.

LACTUCA agnina feu Valerianella foliis ferratis.
R. S. 201.

VALERIANA *Locuſta.* H. F. 12.

Small Corn Sallet, or Valerian with jagged leaves.

In Fields among Corn, and on old Walls —— *common.*
May. A.

LACTUCA fylveſtris murorum. R. S. 162.

PRENANTHES *muralis.* H. F. 296.

Ivy-leaved wild Lettuce.

In Hedges near Wilderton—*uncommon.* July. P.

LACTUCA fylveſtris minima. R. S. 162.

LACTUCA *faligna.* H. F. 296

The leaſt wild Lettuce.

On Banks of Ditches near Sheernefs —— *uncommon.*
Auguſt. A.

LAMIUM album. R. S. 240.

LAMIUM *album* H. F. 225.

White Afchangel or Dead Nettle

Under Hedges — *very common.* May. P.

LAMIUM

LAMIUM rubrum. R. S. 240.
LAMIUM *rubrum.* H. F. 225.
Red Archangel or Dead Nettle.
On Rubbiſh, and ſides of Fields —— very common.
May. A.

LAMIUM cannabinum floribus albis verticillis
purpuraſcentibus. R. S. 241.
GALEOPSIS *Tetrahit.* β. H. F. 226.
White flowered Hemp-leaved Dead Nettle.
In Hedges between Plomford *and* Badgen Downs —
not common. Auguſt. A.

LAMIUM cannabino folio vulgare. R. S. 240.
GALEOPSIS *Tetrahit.* H. F. 226.
Nettle Hemp, or Hemp-leaved Dead Nettle.
In Byſing Wood—*not common.* Auguſt. A.

LAMIUM cannabino folio, flore amplo luteo, labio
purpureo. R. S. 241.
GALEOPSIS *Tetrahit* δ. H. F. 226.
Hemp-leaved Dead Nettle with a parti-coloured
Flower.
In Mr. Jacob's *new Wood-hedge at* Nackington ——
very uncommon. Auguſt. A.

LAMIUM folio caulem ambiente majus ét minus.
R. S. 240.
LAMIUM *amplexicaule.* H. F. 225.
Great Henbit.
In Hop-grounds—very common. June. A.

LAMIUM luteum. R. S. 242.
　GALEOPSIS *Galeobdolon.* H. F. 226.
　Yellow Archangel, Dead Nettle, or yellow Nettle
　　Hemp.
In Woods and under fhady Hedges —— *very common.*
　May. P.

LAMPSANA. R S 173.
　LAPSANA *communis.* H. F. 303.
　Nipple-wort.
In moift Cornfields, and by Way fides—*very common.*
　July. A.

LAPATHUM acetofum repens lanceolatum.
　R. S. 143.
　RUMEX *Acetofella.* H. F. 136.
　Sheep's Sorrel.
On dry fandy or gravelly Ground —— *very common.*
　July. P.

LAPATHUM acetofum vulgare. R. S. 143.
　RUMEX *Acetofa.* H. F. 136.
　Common Sorrel.
In Meadows and Paftures—*very common.* June. B.

LAPATHUM acutum. R. S. 142
　RUMEX *acutus.* H. F. 134.
　Sharp-pointed Dock.
In uncultivated Places—*very common.* June. P.

LAPA-

LAPATHUM acutum minimum. R. S. 141.
An RUMICIS *acuti* varietas. H. F. 134.
The leffer fharp-pointed Dock.
In Woods —— *not uncommon.* June. P.

LAPATHUM folio acuto crifpo. R S. 141.
RUMEX *crifpus* H. F. 134.
Sharp-pointed Dock, with curled Leaves.
On the Mud Walls beyond the Sluice —— *common.*
July. P.

LAPATHUM folio acuto rubente. R. S. 142.
RUMEX *fanguineus.* H. F. 133.
Blood-wort.
In Davington Brooks—*uncommon.* July. B.

LAPATHUM maximum aquaticum five Hydro-
lapathum. R. S. 140.
RUMEX. *Britannica.* H. F. 135.
Great Water Dock.
In Ditches and boggy Places—very common. Auguft. P.

LAPATHUM pulchrum Bononienfe finuatum.
R. S. 142.
RUMEX *pulcher.* H. F. 134.
Fiddle-Dock.
By the fides of Foot-ways about the Town — *not un-*
common. June. P.

LAPATHUM viride. R. S. 141.
   An RUMICIS *acuti* varietas. H. F. 134.
   The greener leaved Dock.
In shady Woods and moist Ground —— not uncommon.
   June. P.

LAPATHUM vulgare folio obtuso. R. S. 141.
   RUMEX *obtusifolius.* H. F. 134.
   Common broad-leaved Dock.
In moist Places, and by Road sides —— very common.
   July. P.

LAPPA major Arctium Dioscoridis. R. S. 197.
   ARCTIUM *Lappa.* H. F. 304.
   Burdock, or Clot burr.
Under Hedges, and by Road-sides —— very common.
   August. B.

LAPPA major capitulo glabro maximo. R.S. 196.
   ARCTIUM *Lappa.* β. H. F. 304.
   Greater Burdock, with a larger Flower.
By Road-sides, and under Hedges —— common.
   August. B.

LAPPA major capitulis parvis glabris. R. S. 197.
   ARCTIUM *Lappa.* H. F. 304.
   Burdock with small Heads.
By Road sides in Hern-hill —— *not uncommon.* August. B.   **LAPPA**

LAPPA major montana capitulis tomentofis.
  ARCTIUM *Lappa.* H. F. 304.
  Greater Burdock with woolly Heads.
In the Way-fides near Luddenham Court—*uncommon.*
  Auguft. B.

LATHYRUS luteus fylveftris dumetorum. R. S.
  320.
  LATHYRUS *pratenfis.* H. F. 277.
  Tare everlafting, or common yellow baftard
  Vetchling.
In Woods and Hedges — *common.* Auguft. A.

LATHYRUS major latifolius. R. S. 319.
  LATHYRUS *latifolius.* H. F. 276.
  Broad-leaved everlafting Pea.
In a Field Hedge at Copton, *and by the Road-fide near*
  Boughton Street—*uncommon.* July. P.

LATHYRI majoris fpecies flore rubente et albido.
  R. S. 319.
  LATHYRUS *fylveftris.* H. F. 276.
  Narrow-leaved everlafting Pea.
In a Hedge of the Beacon Farm—*uncommon.* Au-
  guft. P.

LAUREOLA. R. S. 465.
  DAPHNE *Laureola.*
  Dwarf Laurel, or Spurge-Laurel.
In Woods and under Hedges — *common.* March. P.

LENS paluftris. R. S. 129.

LEMNA *minor*. H. F. 345.

Duck's Meat.

In Ponds and ftanding Waters —— very common.
June. P.

LENTICULA aquatica trifulca. R. S. 129.

LEMNA *trifulca*. H. F. 344.

Ivy-leaved Duck's Meat.

In the Ditches of Ham Marfh—*common.* June. P.

LENTICULA paluftris major. R. S. 129.

LEMNA *polyrhiza*. H. F. 345.

Greater Duck's Meat.

In a Ditch near Waterham—*uncommon.* July. A.

LEPIDIUM latifolium. R. S. 304.

LEPIDIUM *latifolium*. H.F. 244.

Dittander, or Pepperwort.

Near the King's Head Key *in the* Town—*very uncommon.* July. P.

LEUCANTHEMUM vulgare. R. S. 184.

CHRYSANTHEMUM *Leucanthemum*. H. F.
321.

The greater Daifie, or Ox-eye.

In Paftures, and amongft Corn—common. May. P.

LEUCO-

LEUCOJUM luteum vulgo Cheiri flore fimplici.
R. S. 291.
CHEIRANTHUS *Cheiri*. H. F. 250.
Wall-flower, or wild Chier.
On old Walls — very uncommon May. P.

* LEUCOJUM bulbofum trifolium minus.
Bauhini Pinacis. 56.
GALANTHUS *nivalis*. Lin. Syft. Natur.
II. p. 234.
The Snow Prop.
In Paftures at South-ftreet, *and at* Davington ——
very common. February. P.

LIGUSTRUM. R. S. 465.
LIGUSTRUM *vulgare*. H. F. 3.
Privet, or Prim.
In Woods and Hedges — very common. May. S.

LILLIUM convallium. R. S. 264.
CONVALLARIA *majalis*. H. F. 126.
Lilly Convally, or May Lilly.
In the Blean Woods *—plentifully.* May. P.

LIMNOPEUCE. R. S. 136.
HIPPURIS *vulgaris*. H. F. 1.
Mare's Tail.
In the Powder-Mill *Waters—uncommon.* May. P.

LIMONIUM. R. S. 200.
  STATICE *Limonium.* H. F. 114.
  Sea Lavender.
In the Salt Marfhes——very common. Auguft. P.

LINARIA Elatine dicta folio acuminato.
    R. S. * 282.
  ANTIRRHINUM *Elatine.* H. F. 237.
  Sharp po'nted Fluellin.
In Corn Fields — common. September. A.

LINARIA Elatine dicta folio fubrotundo.
    R. S * 282.
  ANTIRRHINUM *fpurium* H F 237.
  Round leaved Fluellin.
- *In the Corn fields of* Prefton—*not uncommon.* Au-
    guft. A

LINARIA lutea vulgaris. R. S. * 281.
  ANTIRRHINUM *Linaria* H F 238.
  Common yellow Toad-flax.
On the fides of Fields and Roads —— very common.
    July. P.

LINUM fylveftre anguftifolium floribus dilute
    purpurafcentibus vel carneis. R. S. 362.
  LINUM *tenuifolium.* H. F. 116.
  Narrow-leaved Wild Flax.
Upon Beacon Hill — *not common.* June. P.

LINUM

LINUM fylveftre cæruleum perenne erectius flore
    et capitulo majore. R. S. 362.
  LINUM *perenne*. H F. 115.
  Perennial Blue Flax.
In the Ifle *of* Shepey — *uncommon*. June. P.

L'NUM fylveftre catharticum. R. S. 362.
  LINUM *catharticum* H. F. 116.
  Purging Flax, Wild Dwarf Flax, Mill-mountain
On fandy and chalky Soils—very common. June. A.

LITHOSPERMUM, feu Milium Solis. R.S. 228.
  LITHOSPERMUM *officinale*. H. F. 65.
  Gromwell, Gromil, or Graymill.
In Badgen Wood, *and by Road fides—not uncommon.*
    June. P.

LONCHITIS afpera. R S. 118.
  OSMUNDA *Spicant*. H. F. 382.
  Rough Spleen-wort.
In the Woods near Dunkirk—*uncommon.* July. P.

LOTI corniculatæ major fpecies. R. S. 334.
  LOTUS *corniculata*. H. F. 288. γ.
  The greater Bird's-foot Trefoil.
Under Hedges near Byfing Wood —— *not common.*
    July. P.

        G   LOTUS

LOTUS corniculata glabra minor. R. S. 334.

LOTUS *corniculata.* H. F. 288.

Bird's-foot Trefoil.

Under Hedges, and in Fields in Ofpringe——*common.*
July. P.

LUPULUS mas et fœmina. R. S. 137.

HUMULUS *Lupulus.* H. F. 369.

Hops, the male and female.

In Hedges in Prefton — *not uncommon.* July. P.

LUTEOLA. R. S. 366.

RESEDA *Luteola.* H. F. 181.

Wild Woad, Yellow Weed, or Dyers Weed.

In Davington *Church-Yard, and on barren Lands —
not uncommon —* June. A.

LYCHNIS major noctiflora Dubrenfis perennis.
R. S. 340.

CUCUBALUS *vifcofus.* H. F. 163.

Dover Campion

On the Cliffs between St Margaret's *and* Dover —
plentifully. July. P.

LYCHNIS maritima repens R S 337.

SILENE *amœna. ?* H F. 164.

Sea Campion

In the Ifle *of* Shepey. — *uncommon.* Auguft P.

LYCH-

LYCHNIS plumaria fylveftris fimplex. R.S. 338.
LYCHNIS *Flos cuculi.* H. F. 174.
Meadow Pink, Wild Williams, Cuckow Flower.
In moift Paftures — very common. June. P.

LYCHNIS Saponaria dicta. R. S. 339.
SAPONARIA *officinalis.* H. F. 160.
Common Soap-wort.
In Hedges near Sindal *and* Keatings, *and beyond*
Sheldwich Church — *uncommon.* July. P.

LYCHNIS fegetum major. R. S. 338.
AGROSTEMMA *Githaco.* H. F. 173.
Cockle.
In Corn Fields — common. June. A.

LYCHNIS fupina maritima Ericæ facie. R.S. 338.
FRANKENIA *lævis.* H. F. 119.
Smooth Sea-Heath.
Near Minfter *in* Shepey—*uncommon.* Auguft. P.

LYCHNIS fylveftris anguftifolia caliculis turgidis
ftriatis R S. 341.
SILENE *conoidea.* H F. 165.
Narrow leaved Campion.
On the Sandhills near Deal — *uncommon.* July.

LYCH-

LYCHNIS fylveftris flore albo. R. S 339.
  LYCHNIS *dioica.* H. F. 174.
  Wild white Campion.
In Woods and Hedges — not uncommon. June. P.

LYCHNIS fylveftris flore rubello. R. S. 339. -
  LYCHNIS *dioica.* H. F. 174. β.
  Red flowered wild Campion.
In Woods and Hedges — common. June. P.

LYCHNIS fylveftris, quæ Behen album vulgo.
    R. S. 337.
  CUCUBALUS *Behen.* H. F. 163.
  Spatling Poppy, Bladder Campion, or white
    Corn Campion.
In dry Paſtures, and in Corn fields—common. July. P.

LYCOPUS paluſtris glaber. R. S. 236.
  LYCOPUS *europæus.* H. F. 8.
  Water Horehound.
On the Banks of the River, and in boggy Places ——
    common. July. P.

LYSIMACHIA campeſtris. R. S. 311.
  EPILOBIUM *montanum.* H. F. 141.
  The greater fmooth-leaved Willow-herb, or
    Loofe-ftrife.
By the fides of Ditches, and under moiſt Hedges ——
    common. July B.   LYSI-

LYSIMACHIA lutea. R. S. 282.

LYSIMACHIA *vulgaris*. H. F. 72.

Yellow Willow-herb, or Loofe-ftrife.

On the fwampy Ground near Stone Bridge — *very un-*
common. Auguft. P.

LYSIMACHIA filiquofa glabra media five minor.
R S. 311.

EPILOBIUM *tetragonum*. H. F. 141.

Middle fmooth-leaved Willow-herb, or Loofe-
ftrife.

In moift Ditches, and near the River — *common*.
July. P.

LYSIMACHIA filiquofa glabra minor anguftifolia R. S. 311

EPILOBIUM *paluftre*. H. F. 141.

The leaft fmooth codded Willow-herb, or Loofe-
ftrife.

In moift Places — *common*. July. P.

LYSIMACHIA filiquofa hirfuta magno flore.
R. S. 311.

EPILOBIUM *ramofum*. H. F. 141.

Great flowered Willow-herb, called Codlings and
Cream.

On the fides of the fhooting Meadow Stream—*common*.
July. P

LYSIMACHIA filiquofa hirfuta parvo flore.
R. S. 311.

EPILOBIUM *hirfutum*. H. F. 140.

The leffer hairy codded Willow-herb, or Loofe-
ftrife.

On the fides of the fhooting Meadow Stream—*common*.
July. P. LYSI-

LYSIMACHIA *fpeciofa*, quibufdam Onagra
dicta. R. S. 310.

EPILOBIUM *anguftifolium*. H. F. 140.
Rofebay Willow-herb.

In a Wood Hedge beyond the five Mile Stone to Charing
— *very uncommon*. July. P.

M.

MALUS fylveftris. R. S. 452.
PYRUS *Malus*. H. F. 189.
The Crab Tree.

In Hedges — *not uncommon*. May. S.

MALVA fylveftris minor. R. S. 251.
MALVA *rotundifolia* H. F. 268.
Small wild or Dwarf Mallow.

On dry Banks by Road fides —— *common*. July to
October. A.

MALVA vulgaris. R. S. 251.
MALVA *fylveftris*. H. F. 268.
Common Mallow.

Under Hedges, by Way fides, and on Rubbifh —— *very
common*. July. B.

MARRUBIUM album. R. S. 239.
MARRUBIUM *vulgare*. H. F. 228.
White Horehound.

On Sheldwich Lees — *not common*. July. P.

MATRI-

MATRICARIA. R. S. 187.

MATRICARIA *Parthenium.* H. F. 321.
Feverfew.
Under Hedges, and on old Walls—common. June P.

MELAMPYRUM fylvaticum flore luteo. R. S.
* 286.
MELAMPYRUM *fylvaticum.* H. F. 236.
Common Cow-wheat with a yellow Flower.
In Byfing Wood*—very common.* June to Auguft. A.

MELILOTUS vulgaris. R. S. 331.
TRIFOLIUM *Melilotus officinalis.* H. F. 282.
Common Melilot.
Amongft the Corn at Halfto*—plentifully.* July B.

* MELISSA officinalis. Miller Botan. Off. 290
MELISSA *officinalis.* Lin. Syftem. Nat. II.
p. 400
Common Garden Balm.
Under Hedges in Boughton *and* Davington —— *un-*
common July. P.

MENIANTHES paluftre triphyllum latifolium
et anguftifolium. R. S. 285.
MENYANTHES *trifolia.* H. F. 71.
Marfh Trefoil, or Buckbean.
In the moift Meadows of the Abbey*—common.* July. P.

MENTHA

MENTHA aquatica feu Syfimbrium   R. S. 233.
   MENTHA *aquatica.* H. F. 223.
   Water-mint.
In moift Places, and by the River fide — very common.
   Auguft. P.

MENTHA feu Calamintha aquatica.   R. S. 232.
   MENTHA *arvenfis.* H F 223.
   Water-mint with whirled coronets.
On the fides of Ditches, and in Corn fields — common.
   Auguft. P.

MENTHA fpicata anguftifolia glabra fpica latiore.
   R. S. 234.
   MENTHA *fpicata.* H. F. 221.
   Spear-mint.
On the Side of the River oppofite the Powder Stove —
   very uncommon. Auguft. P.

MENTHASTRUM folio rugofo rotundiore fpon-
   taneum flore fpicato odore gravi. R. S. 234.
   MENTHA *rotundifolia.* H. F. 221
   Round leaved Horfe-mint
In a Meadow behind King's Mill — *uncommon.* Au-
   guft. P.

MENTHASTRUM fpicatum folio longiore can-
   dicante. R. S. 234.
   MENTHA *longifolia.* H. F. 221.
   Long leaved Horfe-mint.
On the Banks of the River above Ofpringe Church —
   not uncommon. Auguft. P.   MER-

MERCURIALIS annua glabra vulgaris, Mercurialis mas et Foemina. R. S. 139.
MERCURIALIS *annua.* H. F. 371.
French Mercury.
On Rubbifh and in Gardens — not common. September. A.

MERCURIALIS perennis repens. Cynocrambe dicta. R. S. 138.
MERCURIALIS *perennis.* H. F. 371.
Dog's Mercury.
In Woods and under Hedges—very common. April. P.

MESPILUS Apii folio fylveftris fpinofa, five Oxyacantha. R. S. 453.
CRATÆGUS *Oxyacantha.* H. F. 188.
The white Thorn, or Hawthorn, called Quick.
In Woods and Hedges — very common. May. S.

MESPILUS Apii folio fylveftris non fpinofa. R. S. 453.
CRATÆGUS *torminalis.* H. F. 188.
The common or wild Service-tree, or Sorb.
In the Woods about Chart — *uncommon.* April or May. S.

MILLEFOLIUM vulgare. R. S. 183.
ACHILLEA *Millefolium.* H. F. 324.
Common Yarrow, Millfoil, or Nofe-bleed.
In Meadows and Paftures — very common. June. P.

MOL.

MOLLUGO montana minor Gallio albo fimilis.
R. S. 224.
GALIUM *montanum.* H. F. 56.
Small mountain baftard Madder, or mountain
Ladies Bedftraw.
In the Corn fields about Sindal—*not uncommon.* July. P.

MOLLUGO vulgatior. R. S. 223.
GALIUM *Mollugo.* H. F. 56.
Wild Madder, or great baftard Madder.
In Hedges and bufhy Places—very common July. P,

MOLLUGINIS vulgatioris varietas minor.
R. S. 224.
GALIUM *paluftre.* H. F. 57.
White Ladies Bedftraw
On the fides of the fhooting Meadow Stream—*common.*
July. P.

MOSCHATELLINA foliis fumariæ bulbofæ.
R. S. 267.
ADOXA *Mofchatellina.* H. F. 150.
Tuberous Mofchatell.
In Woods and Hedges—very common April. P.

MYOSOTIS fcorpioides hirfuta. R. S. 229.
MYOSOTIS *fcorpioides.* H F. 65.
Moufe-ear Scorpion grafs.
In Woods, on old Walls and dry Paftures——common
April to Auguft. P. MYOSO-

MYOSOTIS fcorpioides paluſtris. R. S. 229.

MYOSOTIS fcorpioides. H. F. 65. δ.

Water Scorpion-grafs.

On the ſides of Ore Mill-pond—*not common.* April
to Auguſt. P.

MYRRHIS fylveſtris feminibus afperis. R. S 220.

SCANDIX *Anthriſcus.* H. F. 108.

Small Hemlock - Chervil with rough Seeds.

Under Hedges, and by the ſides of Ditches —— *common.*
May. A.

N.

NAPUS fylveſtris R. S. 295.

BRASSICA *Napus.* H. F. 253.

Wild Navew

Amongſt Corn, and by the ſides of Ditches——*common.*
May. B.

NARCISSUS fylveſtris pallidus calyce luteo.
R. S. 371.

NARCISSUS *Pſeudo Narciſſus.* H. F. 123.

Wild Englifh Daffodil.

In the Orchards near Selling-Street—*very uncommon.*
April. P.

NASTURTIUM fupinum capfulis verrucofis, five
Coronopus Ruellii R S. 304.

COCHLEARIA *Coronopus.* H. F. 248.

Swine's Crefs

On the ſides of Roads and Foot-paths — *very common.*
July. A. NEPETA

NEPETA major vulgaris. R. S. 237.
  NEPETA *Cataria.* H. F. 220.
  Nep, or Cat-mint.
Under the Weſt Hedge of King's-Field — *not common.*
  July. P.

NUMMULARIA. R. S. 283.
  LYSIMACHIA *Nummularia.* H. F. 73
  Money-wort, or Herb Two-pence
In moiſt Hedges at Luddenham, *and near* Provender
  — not common. June. P.

NUMMULARIA minor flore purpuraſcente.
  R. S 283
  LYSIMACHIA *tenella* H. F 73
  Purple flowered Money-wort.
In moiſt Meadows by the Abbey ——*not uncommon*
  July P

NYMPHÆA alba. R. S. 368.
  NYMPHÆA *alba.* H. F. 206.
  White Water Lilly.
In Ham Ponds *near* Sandwich—*uncommon.* July. P.

NYMPHÆA lutea H F. 368.
  NYMPHÆA *lutea.* H. F 206
  Yellow Water Lilly.
In Ore Mill Pond — *uncommon.* July. P.

OENAN-

O.

OENANTHE *aquatica.* R. S. 210.
　OENANTHE *fiftulofa.* H. F. 104.
　Water Dropwort.
In the Ditches near Fairbrook—*common.* July. P.

OENANTHE Cicutæ facie. Lobellii. R.S. 210.
　OENANTHE *crocata.* H. F. 105.
　Hemlock Dropwort.
In the Water-lane *between* Sitingbourn *and* Milton—
　very uncommon. June. P.

ONOBRYCHIS feu Caput gallinaceum. R S. 327.
　HEDYSARUM *Onobrychis.* H. F. 281.
　Saintfoin or Cock's-head.
On the chalky Hills — *common.* June. P.

OPHIOGLOSSUM. R. S. 128.
　OPH'OGLOSSUM *vulgatum.* H. F. 382.
　Adders Tongue.
In Meadows at Ofpringe *and* Luddenham — *not un-*
　common. May. P.

OPULUS Ruellii. R. S. 4fo.
　VIBURNUM *Opulus.* H. F. 112.
　Water Elder, or Cherrywood.
In Badgen Wood, *and in Hedges* —— *not uncommon.*
　June. S.

H　　　　　　ORCHIS

ORCHIS abortiva rufa five Nidus avis. R. S. 382.
　OPHRYS *Nidus avis.* H. F. 338.
　Birds neft Orchis.
In Byfing *and* Jud's Woods —— *very uncommon.*
　June. P.

ORCHIS alba bifolia minor calcari oblongo.
　　R. S. 380.
　ORCHIS *bifolia.* H. F. 333.
　Butterfly Orchis.
In Badgen *and* Cockfet Woods —— *not common.*
　May. P.

ORCHIS anthropophora oreades. R. S. 397.
　OPHRYS *anthropophora* H F. 340.
　The Green Man Orchis.
On chalky Banks — *common.* June. P.

ORCHIS fuciflora galea et alis purpurafcentibus.
　　R. S. 379.
　OPHRYS *apifera.* H F. 340.
　The Bee Orchis.
In Meadows in Ofpringe—*not uncommon.* June. P.

ORCHIS galea et alis fere cinereis. R. S. 378.
　ORCHIS *militaris.* H. F. 335.
　The Man Orchis.
On chalky bufhy Banks beyond Whitehill, Ofpringe —
　` *not common.* June. P.

　　　　　　　　　　　　　　ORCHIS

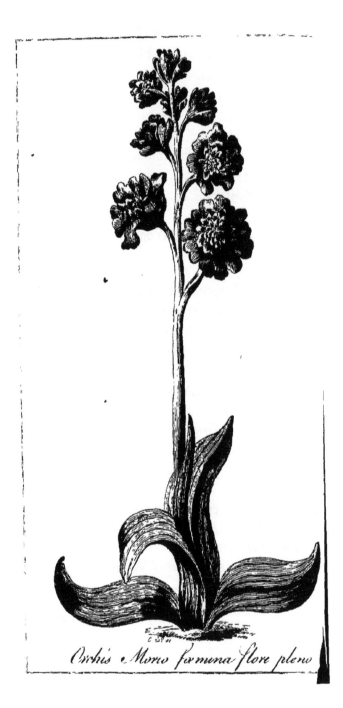

Orchis Morio fœmina flore pleno

ORCHIS magna latifolia galea fufca vel nigricante.
   R S.   378.
   ORCHIS *purpurea*.   H. F.   334.
   The purple Man Orchis.
In Cockfet *and* Jud's Woods—*uncommon*.   May. P.

ORCHIS morio fœmina.   R S.   377.
   ORCHIS *morio*.   H. F.   333.
   Female Orchis, or Female Fools Stones.
*In Meadows —— very common.   In a Meadow neer
   Cades in* Ofpringe, *fome of a Rofe Colour,
   fome white, and a very few with double Flowers.*
   May and June.   P.

ORCHIS morio mas foliis maculatis.   R. S.   376.
   ORCHIS *mafcula*.   H. F.   333.
   Male Orchis, or Male Fools Stones.
In Hedges and Meadows—very common.   May. P.

ORCHIS myodes galea et aliis herbidis.   R.S.   379.
   OPHRYS *mufcifera*.   H. F.   340.
   The Fly Orchis.
Among the Bufhes in Ofpringe Parfonage *Meadows—
   not uncommon.*   June. P.

ORCHIS odorata mofchata.   R. S.   378.
   OPHRYS *Monorchis*.   H. F.   339.
   Yellow or Mufk Orchis.
On the chalky Banks of Ofpringe Parfonage *Mea-
   dows —* uncommon.   June. P.

ORCHIS palmata minor flore luteo-viridi.
R. S. 381.
SATYRIUM *viride*. H. F. 337.
Frog Satyrion or Orchis.
On dry graſſy Banks near Whitehill ——— *uncommon.*
June. P.

ORCHIS palmata pratenſis latifolia longis calca-
ribus. R. S. 380.
ORCHIS *latifolia*. H. F. 335.
Male handed Orchis, or Satyrion royal.
On moiſt boggy Grounds about Ore Mill ——— *not un-*
common. June. P.

ORCHIS palmata ſpecioſiore thyrſo, folio maculato.
R S. 381.
ORCHIS *maculata*. H. F. 335.
Female handed Orchis, or Satyrion royal.
In Chalk Pits — *common.* June. P.

ORCHIS pannonica. R. S. 377.
ORCHIS *uſtulata*. H F. 334.
Little purple flowered Orchis.
On the South ſide of Chatham Hill ——— *plentifully.*
May. P.

ORCHIS purpurea ſpica congeſta pyramidali.
R. S. 377.
· ORCHIS *pyramidalis*. H. F. 334.
Purple late flowering Orchis.
On chalky Banks in Oſpringe — *common.* July. P.

ORCHIS fpiralis alba odorata, five Triorchis.
    R. S. 378.
    OPHRYS *fpiralis.*
    Triple Ladies Traces.
In Ofpringe Parfonage *Meadows* —— *uncommon.*
    September. P.

ORCHIS five Tefticulus fphegodes hirfuto flore.
    R. S. 380.
    OPHRIS *apifera.* H. F. 340. β.
    Humble Bee Orchis with green Wings.
On the Banks of Whitehill *in* Selling —— *uncommon.*
    April. P.

ORIGANUM Onites. R. S. 236.
    ORIGANUM *Onites.* H. F. 229.
    Pot Marjoram.
In Waldeifhare Park—*very uncommon.* Auguft. P.

ORIGANUM vulgare fpontaneum. R. S. 236.
    ORIGANUM *vulgare.* H. F. 229.
    Wild Marjoram.
Under Hedges, and in bufhy Places —— *very common.*
    July. P.

ORNITHOPODIUM radice nodofa. R. S. 326.
    ORNITHOPUS *perpufillus.* H. F. 280.
    Birds Foot.
In Broom fields at Hernhill—*common.* May to Au-
    guft. P.

ORABAN-

OROBANCHE major Garyophyllum olens.
R. S. * 288.
OROBANCHE *major*. H. F. 232.
Broom-rape.
In Broom fields — not uncommon. June. B.

OROBUS fylvaticus foliis oblongis glabri*.
R. S. 324.
OROBUS *tuberofus*. H. F. 274.
Wood Pea, or Heath Pea.
In Jud's Wood *— very common.* May. P.

OSTRYA Ulmo fimilis, fructu in umbilicis foliaceis.
R. S. 451.
CARPINUS. *Betulus*. H. F. 360.
The Horn-beam Tree, or Horfe-Beech.
In Woods — common. May. S.

OXYS alba. R. S. * 281.
OXALIS *Acetofella*. H. F. 173.
Wood Sorrel.
In Byfing *and* Jud's Woods *— common.* June. A.

P.

PAPAVER corniculatum luteum. R. S. 309.
CHELIDONIUM *Glaucium*. H. F. 202.
Yellow horned Poppy.
On the Beach at Sea-Salter *— common.* July. A.

PAPAVER

PAPAVER corniculatum luteum. Chelidonia
    dictum. R. S 309.
CHELIDONIUM *majus*. H. F. 201.
The greater Celandine.
Among Rubbish, and on old Walls—common. June. P.

PAPAVER laciniato folio capitulo breviore glabro
    annuum, Rhœas dictum. R. S. 308.
PAPAVER *Rhæas*. H. F. 203.
Red Poppy, or Corn Poppy.
In Corn fields — very common. July. A.

PARIETARIA. R. S. 158.
PARIETARIA *officinalis*. H. F. 376.
Pellitory of the Wall.
On old Walls — very common. July. P.

PARONYCHIA vulgaris. R. S. 292.
DRABA *verna*. H. F. 243.
Common Whitlow Grafs.
On old Walls and dry Pastures —— very common.
    April. A.

PASTINACA fylveftris latifolia. R. S. 206.
PASTINACA *fativa*. H. F. 109.
Wild Parfnep.
On the chalky Bank by the Roadfide near Wilderton—
    uncommon. July. B.

PEDI-

PEDICULARIS feu Crifta galli lutea. R. S.
  * 284.

RHINANTHUS *Crifta galli.* H. F. 234.
Yellow Rattle, or Cocks-comb.

In Byfing Wood *, and by Road fides—common.* July. A.

PEDICULARIS paluftris rubra elatior. R. S.
  * 284.

PEDICULARIS *paluftris.* H. F. 236.
Great Marfh red Rattle, Cocks-comb, Loufe-
wort.

About the Powder Mills *at* Ore—*not common.* June. A.

PEDICULARIS pratenfis rubra vulgaris. R. S.
  * 284.

PEDICULARIS *fylvatica.* H. F. 236.
Red Rattle, Cocks-comb, Loufe-wort.

In Jud's Wood — *common.* June. P.

PENTAPHYLLOIDES Argentina dicta. R. S.
  256.

POTENTILLA *Argentina.* H. F. 195.
Wild Tanfey, or Silver-weed.

By the fides of Roads and Paths—common. July. P.

PENTAPHYLLUM erectum foliis profunde
  fectis fubtus argenteis flore luteo. R. S 255.
POTENTILLA *argentea.* H. F. 196.
Tormentil Cinquefoil.

In a Read hedge near Newnham.—*uncommon.* May. P
                                            PENTA-

PENTAPHYLLUM vulgatiffimum. R. S. 225.
POTENTILLA *reptans*. H. F. 197.
Common Cinquefoil, or Five-fingered Grafs.
By the fides of Roads and Paths—common. June. P.

PENTAPTEROPHYLLON aquaticum, flofculis
ad foliorum nodos. R. S. 316.
MYRIOPHYLLUM *verticillatum.* H. F. 357.
Verticillated Water-millfoil.
In the Ditches of Graveney Marfh — *not uncommon.*
July. P.

PERCEPIER Anglorum. R. S. 159.
APHANES *arvenfis.* H. F. 60.
Purfley-piért.
Upon barren Lands and old Walls—common. May. A.

PERSICARIA latifolia geniculata caulibus macu-
latis. R. S. 145.
POLYGONUM *Perficaria*. H. F. 147. β.
Dead or fpotted Arfmart.
In Fields, and on Rubbifh — common. Auguft. A.

PERSICARIA maculofa. R. S. 145.
POLYGONUM *Perficaria*. H. F. 147.
Dead or fpotted Arfmart.
In Meadows and Ditches—very common. Sept. A.

PERSI-

PERSICARIA mitis major foliis pallidioribus.
R. S. 145.
POLYGONUM *penfylvanicum.* H. F. 148.
Greater dead Arfmart with pale Leaves.
On a Dunghill at Staple Street —— *uncommon.*
Auguft. A.

PERSICARIA falicis folio perennis, Potamogiton
anguftifolium dicta. R. S. 145.
POLYGONUM *amphibium.* H. F. 147.
Perennial Willow-leaved Arfmart.
On the fides of the Abby Ditches —— *not common.*
July. P.

PERSICARIA vulgaris acris, feu Hydropiper.
R. S. 144.
POLYGONUM *Hydropiper.* H. F. 148.
Lakeweed, Arfmart, Water-pepper.
In moift Places and wet Ditches —— *very common*
Auguft. A.

PETASITES. R. S. 179.
TUSSILAGO *Petafites.* H. F. 315.
Common Butter Bur, Peftilent-wort.
Near Waterham *in* Hernhill—*uncommon.* March. P.

* PETROSELINUM vulgare. Miller. Botan.
Officinal. 324.
APIUM *Petrofelinum.* Linnæi Syftem. Natur.
II. p. 217.
Common Parfley.
On the Weft Church-yard Wall —— *very uncommon.*
June. B.   PEU-

PEUCEDANUM. R. S. 206.

PEUCEDANUM *officinale*. H. F. 101.
Hog-fennel, or Sulphur-wort.

On the Wall leading to Thorn Creek —— *plentifully*.
June. P.

PHELLANDRIUM vel Cicutaria aquatica quorundam. R. S. 215.

PHELLANDRIUM *aquaticum*. H. F. 107.
Water Hemlock.

On boggy Ground between Staple-Street *and* Hernhill Church — *uncommon*. July. B.

PHYLLITIS feu Lingua cervina vulgo. R. S. 116.

ASPLENIUM *Scolopendrium*. H. F. 384.
Hart's Tongue.

*In fhady Lanes, hollow Ways, and on Walls——com-
mon*. P.

PILOSELLA repens. R. S 170.

HIERACIUM *Pilofella* H F. 298.
Common creeping Moufe ear.

On dry fandy Banks — *common*. May. A.

PIMPINELLA Saxifraga R. S. 213.

PIMPINELLA *major*. H. F. 110.
Great Burnet-faxifrage.

In a thick Hedge beyond Whitehill —— *uncommon*.
Auguft. P.

PIMPI-

PIMPINELLA Saxifraga minor. R. S. 213.
PIMPINELLA *Saxifraga.* H. F. 111. β.
Small Burnet-faxifrage with divided Leaves.
In Meadows in Hernhill —— *not uncommon.* August. P.

PIMPINELLA Saxifraga minor foliis fanguiforbæ. R. S. 213.
PIMPINELLA *Saxifraga.* H. F. 111.
The leffer round leaved Burnet-faxifrage.
In dry Paftures —— *common.* Auguft and September. P.

PLANTAGO aquatica. R. S. 257.
ALISMA *Plantago.* H. F. 137.
Great Water Plantain.
In moift Places, and on the fides of Ponds —— *common.* Auguft. P.

PLANTAGO foliis laciniatis, Coronopus dicta.
PLANTAGO *Coronopus.* H. F. 52.
Buck's-horn Plantain, Star of the Earth.
In the Abby Meadows —*very common.* Auguft. A.

PLANTAGO latifolia vulgaris. R. S. 314.
PLANTAGO *major* H. F. 51.
Great Plantain, Way-bread.
By Way fides —— *very common.* July. P. The Plantago panicula fparfa, found in *Perry field,* is an elegant variety of this Plant, but very uncommon. PLAN-

PLANTAGO major incana. R S 314.
  PLANTAGO *media*. H. F. 51.
  Hoary Plantain.
By Road sides — common. July. P.

PLANTAGO marina. R S. 315.
  PLANTAGO *Loeflingii.* H. F. 52.
  Sea Plantain.
On the sides of the Ditches and Sea Walls —common.
      July. P.

PLANTAGO *maritima.* H. F. 52.
  Narrow leaved Plantain.
In the Brent Marshes—*not uncommon.* July. P.

PLANTAGO quinquenervia. R. S. 314.
  PLANTAGO *lanceolata.* H. F. 52.
  Rib-wort, or Rib wort Plantain.
In Fields and Meadows —— very common. June to
      August. P.

POLYGALA R. S. * 287.
  POLYGALA *vulgaris.* H. F. 271.
  Milk-wort.
In dry Fields, and under Hedges—— very common.
      June. P.

I   POLY-

POLYGONUM brevi anguſtoque folio. R.S 146
   POLYGONUM *aviculare.* H F 149. β.
   Knot-graſs with a ſmall narrow Leaf.
By Road ſides—common. June to September A

POLYGONUM mas vulgare R S. 146.
   POLYGONUM *aviculare.* H. F. 149.
   Common Knot-graſs.
In uncultivated Ground, and by Way ſides —— *very*
   common. June to October. A.

POLYGONUM oblongo anguſtoque folio.
   R S. 146
   POLYGONUM *aviculare* H F 149. γ.
   Knot-graſs with a more oblong narrow Leaf.
In Corn fields at Hernhill — *common* June to Sep-
   tember. A.

POLYPODIUM. R. S. 117.
   POLYPODIUM *vulgare* H F. 387
   Common Polypody.
In Byfing Wood, *and on Banks of ho'ow Ways* ——
   common. P.

POPULAGO, ſive Caltha paluſtris R S. 272.
   CALTHA *paluſtris.* H. F. 214.
   Marſh Marigold.
In the Brent Marſhes—*very common.* April. P.

POPULUS alba. R. S. 446.
POPULUS *alba*. H. F. 370.
The White Poplar, or Abele Tree.
In m ift Woods, and boggy Places —— *common.*
March. S.

POPULUS I ybica Plinii. R. S. 446.
POPULUS *tremula*. H. F. 370.
The Afp, or Trembling Poplar.
In moift Places in Hernhill —— *not uncommon.*
March. S.

POPULUS major R. S. 446.
POPULUS *nigra*. H F. 370.
The Black Poplar.
In moift boggy Places in Hernhill — *not uncommor.*
March S.

PORTULA. R S. 368.
PEPLIS *Portulaca*. H. F. 128.
Water Purflane.
In the Brent Meadows — *not uncommon.* September
ber P

POTAMOGITON foliis pennatis. R S. 150.
MYRIOPHYLLUM *fpicatum*. H F. 357.
Feathered or fpiked Water Millfoil
In the Powder Mill *Waters*, and Graveney Marfh
Dykes — *common.* July. P.

POTA-

POTAMOGITON feu Fontalis crifpa. Tribulus
    aquaticus. R. S. 149.
  POTAMOGETON *crifpum.* H. F. 61.
The greater Water Caltrops
In the Powder Mill Waters—*common* June P.

POTAMOGETON feu Fontalis media lucens.
  R S. 149
  POTAMOGETON *ferratum.* H. F 64.
The leffer Water Caltrops, or Frog's Lettuce.
In the River near the Powder Stove—*not uncommon.*
  June. P.

POTAMOGITON gramineum latiufculum foliis
    èt ramificationibus denfe ftipatis. R S. 149.
  POTAMOGETON *gramineum.* H. F. 62.
Grafs leaved Pond weed.
In the fhallow Waters about the Powder Mills — *not
  common.* P.

POTAMOGITON maritimu n ramofiffimum gran-
    diufculis capitulis, capillaceo folio noftras.
    R.S. 150.
  POTAMOGETON *marinum.* H. F. 63.
Sea Pond-weed.
In Dykes near Sheernefs — *uncommon.* Auguft. P.

POTAMOGITON millefolium, feu foliis gramineis
    ramofum. R. S. 150.
  POTAMOGETON *pectinatum.* H. F. 62.
Fine or Fennel-leaved Pond-weed.
In Ofpringe River — *not common.* June. P.

POTAMOGITON perfoliatum. R. S. 149.
  POTAMOGETON *perfoliatum.* H. F. 60.
  Perfoliated Pond-weed.
In Ofpringe River — *common.* July. P.

POTAMOGITON rotundifolium. R. S. 148.
  POTAMOGETON *natans.* H. F. 60.
  Broad leaved Pond-weed.
In a Pond near Uplees — *uncommon.* Auguft. P.

PRIMULA pratenfis inodora lutea. R. S. 284.
  PRIMULA *veris* H F. 70. β.
  Great Cowflips, or Oxflips.
In thick Hedges beyond Whitehill — *not common.*
  April. P.

PRIMULA veris major. R. S. 284.
  PRIMULA *veris.* H. F. 71. α.
  Common Pagils, or Cowflips.
In Meadows and Hedges—very common. April. P.

PRIMULA veris vulgaris. R. S. 284.
  PRIMULA *vulgaris.* H. F. 70.
  Common Primrofe.
In Woods and Hedges — very common. February to
  May. P.

PRUNELLA. R. S. 238.
  PRUNELLA *vulgaris*. H. F. 231.
  Common Self-heal.
In Meadows — common. Auguft. P.

PRUNUS fylveftris. R. S. 48.
  PRUNUS *fpinofa.* H. F. 186.
  The Black Thorn, or Sloe Tree.
In Hedges — very common. April. S.

PRUNUS fylveftris major. R. S. 462.
  PRUNUS *infititia.* H F. 186.
  The black Bullace Tree.
In fome Hedges near Rickefey-Lane *in* Selling ——
  uncommon. April. S.

PRUNUS fylveftris fruftu majore albo. R.S. 462.
  PRUNUS *infititia.* H. F. 186. γ.
  The white Bullace Tree.
In Hedges at Cades *in* Ofpringe, *and at* Selling —
  uncommon. April. S.

PRUNUS fylveftris fruftu rubro acerbo et ingrato.
  R. S. 463.
PRUNUS *infititia.* H. F. 186. β.
  The Scad Tree.
In Hedges — not uncommon. April. S.

PTAR-

PTARMICA. R. S. 183.

ACHILLEA *Ptarmica*. H. F. 325.

Sneeze-wort, Baftard Pellitory, or Goofe-tongue.

In Davington Brooks — *uncommon.* Auguft. P.

PULEGIUM. R. S 235.

MENTHA *Pulegium.* H. F. 224.

Penny-royal, or Pudding-grafs.

In a fmall Pond at Elvyland *in* Ofpringe—*uncommon.*

PYRASTER feu Pyrus fylveftris. R. S. 452.

PYRUS *communis.* H. F. 189.

The Wild Pear Tree.

In the Wood leading from Keneways *to* Wilderton —
  very uncommon. April. S.

Q.

QUERCUS latifolia. R. S. 440.

QUERCUS *Robur.* H. F. 359.

The common Oak Tree.

In Woods—very common. April. P.

QUERCUS latifolia mas quæ brevi pediculo eft.
  R. S. 440.

QUERCUS *Robur.* H. F. 359. β.

The Oak Tree.

In Woods and Hedges—common. April. S.

RADI-

R.

RADICULA fylveftris feu paluftris. R. S. 301.
SISYMBRIUM *amphibium*. H. F. 258. α.
Water Radifh.

About the Powder-Mill Waters —— *not common.*
June. P.

RADIOLA vulgaris ferpyllifolia Millegrana'
minima. R. S 345
LINUM *Radiola*. H. F. 117.
The leaft Rupture-wort, or All-feed.

On fandy Banks between Ore *and* Luddenham ——
common. A.

RANUNCULO five Polyanthemo aquatili albo
affine. R. S. 250.
RANUNCULUS *aquatilis*. H. F. 213. γ.
Fennel-leaved Crow-foot.

In Running Waters — *common.* May. P.

RANUNCULUS aquaticus albus, circinatis
tenuiffime divifis foliis, floribus ex alis longis
pediculis innixis. R. S. 249.
RANUNCULUS *aquatilis*. H. F. 213. δ.
Fineft leaved Water Crow-foot.

In the Brent Dykes — *common.* April to June. P.

RANUN-

RANUNCULUS aquatilis. R. S. 249.
  RANUNCULUS *aquatilis.* H. F. 213.
  Various leaved Water Crow-foot.
In the fhooting Meadow Stream —— *common.*
  May. P.

RANUNCULUS aquatilis hederaceus albus.
  R. S 249.
  RANUNCULUS *hederaceus.* H. F. 212.
  Ivy leaved Water Crow-foot.
By the Wall that leads to Thorn—*common.* May. P.

RANUNCULUS aquatilis omnino tenuifolius.
  R. S. 249.
  RANUNCULUS *aquatilis.* H. F. 213. β.
  Fine leaved Water Crow-foot.
In Cfpringe River *near* Whitehill—*common.* April
  to June. P.

RANUNCULUS arvorum. R. S. 248.
  RANUNCULUS *arvenfis.* H. F. 212.
  Corn Crow-foot.
In Corn fields—*very common.* June. A.

RANUNCULUS bulbofus. R. S. 247.
  RANUNCULUS *bulbofus.* H F. 211.
  Round rooted or bulbous Crow-foot, or Butter-
  cups
In Meadows — *very common.* May. P.

                                         RANUN-

RANUNCULUS flammeus major. R S 250.
RANUNCULUS *Lingua*. H. F. 210.
Great Spear-wort.

In the old Haven near Sandwich —— *very uncommon.*
May. P.

RANUNCULUS flammeus minor. R S. 250.
RANUNCULUS *Flammula*. H.F. 210.
The leſſer Spear-wort.

In the ſhooting Meadow Stream—*common.* June to
September. P.

RANUNCULUS nemoroſus dulcis ſecundus
Tragi. R. S. 248.
RANUNCULUS *Auricomus*. H F 211.
Sweet wood Crow-foot, or Goldilocks.

In Woods and under Hedges—*common.* April. P.

RANUNCULUS paluſtris. R. S. 249
RANUNCULUS *ſceleratus*. H. F. 212.
Round leaved Water Crow-foot.

On the Banks of the Brent Marſhes —— *common.*
June. A.

RANUNCULUS pratenſis erectus acris. R. S.
248.
RANUNCULUS *acris*. H F. 211.
Upright Meadow Crow foot.

In Meadows —— *very common.* June. P.

RANUNCULUS pratenſis repens R S. 247.
RANUNCULUS *repens*. H. F 210
Common creeping Crow foot.

On Beacon Hill — *common.* May. P.

RAPA

RAPA fativa rotunda. R. S. 294.
  BRASSICA *Rapa*. H. F. 253.
  Turneps.
In Corn fields, and by Way fides —— *not uncommon.*
  April. B.

RAPISTRUM arvorum. R. S. 295.
  SINAPIS *arvenfis*. H. F. 260.
  Charlock, or Wild Muftaid.
In Fields among Corn—common. May. A.

RAPISTRUM floie luteo, filiqua glabra articulata.
  R S 296.
  RHAPHANUS *Rhaphaniftrum*. H.F. 252. β.
  Yellow flowered Charlock with a jointed Cod.
In Fields among Corn — common. July A

RAPUNCULUS Scabiofæ capitulo cæiuleo.
  R. S. 278.
  JASIONE *montana* H. F. 329.
  Hairy Sheep's Scabious.
By the Way fides near Dunkirk —— *uncommon.*
  Auguft. A.

RESEDA vulgaris. R. S. 366.
  RESEDA *lutea*. H. F. 181.
  Bafe Rocket.
In Boughton Chalk Pits — *not common.* July. A.

RHAM-

RHAMNOIDES fructifera, foliis Salicis, baccis leviter flavescentibus. R. S 445.
HIPPOPHAE *Rhamnoides.* H. F. 368.
Sea Buck Thorn, or Sallow Thorn.
In Shepey, *uncommon; near* Sandown Castle — *plentifully.* April. S.

RHAMNUS catharticus. R S. 466.
RHAMNUS *catharticus.* H. F. 83.
Buck Thorn, or Purging Thorn.
In Perry Wood *and* Badgen Down *Hedges — not common* May. S.

RHAPHANISTRUM siliqua articulata glabra majore et minore. R S 296
RHAPHANUS *Rhaphanistrum.* H. F. 252.
White flowered Charlock with a jointed Cod.
In Fields among Corn —— common. June. A.

RHAPHANUS rusticanus. R. S. 301.
COCHLEARIA *Armoracia.* H F. 248.
Horse Radish
On the Banks of the River, *above the* Sluice, *and of* Ore Stream—*uncommon.* June. P.

RIBES nigrum vulgo dictum folio olente. R.S. 456.
RIBES *nigrum.* H. F. 85.
Black Currants, or Squinancy Berries.
In the boggy Osier Ground near Stone Bridge — *uncommon.* May. S.　　　　　RIBES

* RIBES vulgare fructu rubro. R. S. 465.

   RIBES *rubrum.* H. F. 84.

   Currants.

In some thick Hedges in Ospringe —— *not common.*

   May. S.

ROSA sylvestris altera minor, flore albo nostras.

   R. S. 455.

   ROSA *arvensis.* H. F. 192.

   White flowered Dog's Rose.

In Hedges —— very common June. S.

ROSA sylvestris inodora seu canina. R. S. 454.

   ROSA *canina.* H. F. 192.

   Red flowered wild Dog's Rose, or Hep Tree.

In Hedges — very common. June. S.

* ROSA sylvestris odora. R S. 454.

   ROSA *Eglanteria.* H. F. 191.

   Sweet Briar.

In a Hedge near Ore Stray ——*very uncommon.*

   June. S.

ROSA pumila spinosissima, foliis Pimpinellæ

   glabris flore albo. R. S. 455.

   ROSA *spinosissima.* H. F. 191.

   The Burnet Rose.

On the North side of Chatham Hill —— *uncommon.*

   June. S.

           K   RUBE-

RUBEOLA arvenfis repens cærulea. R. S. 225.
SHERARDIA *arvenfis* H F. 54.
Little Field Madder.

In Cades *new Wood, and in Broom fields in* Hernhill — *not uncommon.* May. A.

RUBEOLA vulgaris quadrifolia lævis floribus
purpurafcentibus. R. S. 225.
ASPERULA *Cynanchica.* H F. 55.
Squinancy Wort.

In Ofpringe *Chalk Pits, and on* Badgen Down ——
July. P.

RUBUS Idæus fpinofus fructu rubro R S 467.
RUBUS *Idæus.* H. F. 193
The Rafpberry Bufh.

In Stocking Wood, *near* Lees Court, *and in* Perry
Wood — *not common* May S

RUBUS major fructu nigro R. S 467
RUBUS *fruticofus.* H F. 193.
The Bramble, or Blackberry Bufh.

In Woods and Hedges — very common. June S.

RUBUS minor fructu cæruleo. R. S 467.
RUBUS *cæfius.* H F. 193
The fmall Bramble, or Dew-berry Bufh.

In Woods and Hedges — common. July. S.

RUSCUS.

RUSCUS. R. S. 262.
RUSCUS *aculeatus.* H F. 373.
Knee Holly, or Butcher's broom.
In Ofpringe *Woods and Hedges—common.* April. P.

RUTA *muraria.* R S. 122.
ASPLENIUM *Ruta muraria.* H F. 386.
Wall Rue, White Maiden-hair, Tentwort.
On the Buttrices near the South Door of the Church —
very uncommon P.

S.

SALICARIA vulgaris purpurea foliis oblongis.
R. S 367.
LYTHRUM *Salicaria.* H. F. 179.
Purple-fpiked Loofeftrife, or Willow herb
In the fwampy Ground near Stone-bridge — *not un-
common.* Auguft. P.

SALICORNIA geniculata annua. R. S. 136.
SALICORNIA *europæa.* H. F. 1.
Marfh Sampire, Jointed Glafs-wort, or Salt-wort.
In the Marfhes as you go to Thorn — *common.* Au-
guft. A.

SALIX. R. S. 447.
SALIX *alba.* H. F. 366.
The common white Willow.
In moift Places about the Powder Mills—*not common.*
April. S.   SALIX

SALIX folio articulato fplendente flexilis. R. S.
448.

SALIX *amygdalina*. H. F. 363.

The round eared fhining Willow, or Almond-
leaved Willow.

In a Hedge as you enter Sheldwich Road—*uncommon.*
May. S.

SALIX folio longiffimo. R. S. 450.

SALIX *vimenalis*. H F 366.

The Ofier.

In moift Places — common. April. S.

SALIX latifolia rotunda. R. S. 449.

SALIX *capræa*. H. F. 366.

The common round-leaved Sallow.

In Woods and Hedges — common. April. S.

SALIX pumila foliis utrinque candicantibus et
lanuginofis. R. S. 447.

SALIX *arenaria*. H. F. 364.

Sand Willow.

On the Sand Downs near Deal—*plentifully* June. S.

SAMBUCUS. R. S. 461.

SAMBUCUS *nigra*. H F. 112.

Common Elder

In Hedges — very common May. S.

SAMBU-

SAMBUCUS humilis, feu Ebulus. R. S. 461.
  SAMBUCUS *Ebulus*. H. F. 113.
Dwarf Elder, Wall-wort, or Dane-wort.
By the Road fides near Boughton-Street ——*not un-
  common*. July. P.

SAMOLUS Valerandi. R. S. 283.
  SAMOLUS *Valerandi*. H F. 79.
Round-leaved Water Pimpernel.
In the Brent Marfhes — *common*. June. P.

SANGUISORBA minor R. S. 203.
POTERIUM *Sanguiforba*. H. F. 358.
  Burnet.
On the chalky Hills in Ofpringe—*common*. July. P.

SANICULA five Diapenfia R S. 221.
  SANICULA *europæa*. H F 96.
  Sanicle
In Woods — *very common*. May. P.

SAXIFRAGA aurea. R. S. 158.
  CHRYSOSPLENIUM *oppofitifolium*. H. F.
    156.
  Golden Saxifrage
In Jud's Wood — *not common*. April. P.

SAXIFRAGA rotundifolia alba. R. S. 354.
SAXIFRAGA *granulata.* H. F. 159.
White Saxifrage, or Sen-green.
Upon Beacon Hill — *uncommon.* May. P.

SAXIFRAGA verna annua. R. S. 354.
SAXIFRAGA *tridactylites.* H. F. 159.
Rue-leaved Saxifrage, or Whitlow-grafs.
On Houfes and Walls — very common. April. A.

SCABIOSA major communior folio lacinrato.
R. S. 191.
SCABIOSA *arvenfis.* H F. 50.
Common Field Scabious.
In moift Fields among Corn, and on Bank fides—com-
mon. Auguft. P. With a proliferous Flower
in *Badgen Wood,* uncommon.

SCABIOSA minor vulgaris R. S 191.
SCABIOSA *Columbaria.* H. F. 50.
The lefler Field Scabious.
In dry hilly Places — not uncommon. July P.

SCABIOSA radice fuccifa, flore globofo. R.S. 191.
SCABIOSA *Succifa.* H. F. 50.
Devil's Bit.
In Byfing Wood *and the* Abby Meadows—*common.*
Auguft. P.

SCAN-

SCANDIX femine roftrato vulgaris. R. S. 207.
  SCANDIX *Pecten Veneris.* H. F. 107.
  Shepherd's Needle, or Venus Comb.
In Fields among Corn—very common. July. A.

SCORODONIA feu Salvia agreftis. R S. 245.
  TEUCRIUM. *Scorodonia.* H. F. 219.
  Wood Sage.
In Byfing Wood *— very common.* July. P.

SCROPHULARIA aquatica major. R S. * 283.
  SCROPHULARIA *aquatica* H. F. 239.
  Water Betony, Water Figwort.
On the Banks of the River, *and in moift Ditches——
    common.* July. P.

SCROPHULARIA major. R. S. * 283.
  SCROPHULARIA *nodofa.* H. F 239.
  Common knobby-rooted Figwort.
In moift Hedges — common. July. P.

SEDUM minimum non acre flore albo. R. S.
    270.
  SEDUM *annuum.* H. F. 172.
  Mountain Stone-crop.
On the Beach near Sandown Caftle —— *plentifully.*
    Auguft. P.

SEDUM minus hæmatoides. R. S. 269.
, SEDUM *reflexum*. H. F. 170. β.
Yellow Stone-crop, or Prick-madam.
On the Abby Walls — *common.* July. P.

SEDUM minus luteum ramulis reflexis. R. S.
270.
SEDUM *reflexum* H. F. 170.
Yellow reflexed Stone-crop.
On the Abby Walls — *common* July. P.

SEDUM parvum acre flore luteo. ' R. S. 270.
SEDUM *acre.* H. F. 171.
Stone-crop, or Wall-pepper.
On Walls and Houses — *not uncommon.* July. P.

SEDUM *sexangulare.* H. F. 171.
Infipid Stone-crop.
Near Sheernefs —— *plentifully* July. B.

SEMPERVIVUM majus. R. S. 269.
SEMPERVIVUM *tectorum.* H. F. 185.
Houfe-leek, or Sengreen.
On Walls and tiling of Houfes —— *not uncommon.*
July. P.

SENECIO

SENECIO vulgaris. R. S. 178.
   SENECIO vulgaris. H. F. 315.
   Common Groundfel, or Simfon.
In Fields and under Hedges ——— very common.
   May. A.

SERPYLLUM citratum. R. S. 230.
   THYMUS *Serpyllum.* H. F. 229 ε.
   Lemon Thyme.
On Badgen Down *— not common.* July. P.

SERPYLLUM vulgare. R. S. 230.
   THYMUS *Serpyllum.* H. F. 229.
   Mother of Thyme.
On dry billy Ground —— very common. July. P.

SERRATULA. R. S. 196.
   SERRATULA *tinctoria.* H. F. 304.
   Saw-wort.
Near the late Decoy Ponds at Graveney—*uncommon.*
   July. P.

SESELI pratenfe noftras. R. S. 216.
   SESELI *Caruifolia.* H. F. 106.
   Meadow Saxifrage.
In the low Meadows in Hernhill, *and in* Shepey ——
   not uncommon. Auguft. P.

SIDERI-

SIDERITIS anglica ftrumofa radice. R. S. 242.
STACHYS *paluftris*. H. F. 227.
Clowns Allheal.
In moift Places, and near the River —— *common.*
Auguft. P.

SIDERITIS arvenfis rubra. R. S. 242.
GALEOPSIS *Ladanum.* H. F. 225.
Narrow leaved Allheal, or Iron-wort.
In Ofpringe *Corn fields* — *common.* Auguft. A.

SIDERITIS humilis lato obtufo folio R. S 242.
GLECHOMA *arvenfis.* H. F. 224.
Upright Ground Ivy.
In Ore *Corn fields* —— *common.* Auguft. A.

* SINAPI album fil;qua hirfuta, femine albo vel
ruffo. R. S. 295.
SINAPIS *alba.* H F. 260.
White Muftard.
By the Way fide in the Brent Marfh—*very uncommon.*
Auguft. A.

SINAPI fativum fecundum. R. S. 295.
SINAPIS *nigra.* H. F. 260.
Common Muftard.
In Shepey *amongft Corn, and by Way fides* — *plenti-*
fully. July. A.

SISYM-

SISYMBRIUM Cardamine feu Nafturtium aqua-
    ticum   R. S. 300.
    SISYMBRIUM *Nafturtium.*
    Water Crefs.
By the River fides — very common. July. B. or P.

SISYMBRIUM hirfutum. R. S. 233.
    MENTHA *aquatica.* H F. 223. γ.
    Water Mint
On the fides of the River *— very common.* July. P.

SIUM aromaticum. Sifon officinarum. R S 211.
    SISON *Amomum.* H. F. 104.
    Baftard Stone Parfley.
In a Hedge near Thorn —— *not uncommon.* Au-
    guft. P.

SIUM arvenfe five fegetum. R. S. 211.
    SISON *fegetum.* H. F. 104.
    Corn Parfley, or Honewort.
In moift Hedges near Ewell —— *not uncommon.*
    July. B.

SIUM latifolium foliis variis. R. S. 211.
    SIUM *latifolium.* H. F. 103.
    Great Water Paifnep.
In marfhy Ground, and by the River fide —— *common.*
    Auguft. P.

                             SIUM

SIUM pufillum foliis variis. R. S. 212.
  SISON *inundatum.* H. F. 104.
  The leaft Water Parfnep.
In the Dykes of Nagden Marfh —— *not common.*
    June. A.

SIUM umbellatum repens. R. S. 211.
  SIUM *nodiflorum.* H. F. 103.
  Creeping Water Parfnep.
In the Abby *Ditches* —— *common.* Auguft. P.

SMYRNIUM. R. S. 208.
  SMYRNIUM *Olufatrum.* H. F. 109.
  Alexanders.
In a Hedge as you enter Graveney Marfh—*uncommon.*
    June. B,

SOLANUM lignofum feu Dulcamara. R.S. 255.
  SOLANUM *Dulcamara.* H. F. 78.
  Woody Night-fhade, or Bitter-fweet.
In moift Woods and Hedges— *common.* July. P.

* SOLANUM pomo fpinofo oblongo flore cala-
    thoide, Stramonium vulgo dictum. R.S. 266.
  DATURA *Stramonium..* H. F. 78,
  Thorn Apple.
On Dunghills — *very uncommon.* Auguft. A.

SOLANUM vulgare. R. S. 265.
SOLANUM *nigrum.* H. F. 78.
Common Night-fhade.
On Rubbifh and Dungbills — very common. July. A.

SONCHUS afper laciniatus. R. S. 163.
SONCHUS *oleraceus.* H. F. 294. γ.
Prickly Sow-thiftle with jagged Leaves.
On Rubbifh and in cultivated Grounds —— *common.*
Auguft. A.

SONCHUS afper non laciniatus. R. S. 163.
SONCHUS *oleraceus.* H. F. 294. δ.
Prickly Sow-thiftle with lefs jagged Leaves.
In cultivated Grounds, and on Rubbifh —— *common.*
June to Auguft. A.

SONCHUS lævis. R S. 162.
SONCHUS *oleraceus.* H. F. 294. α.
Common Sow-thiftle.
On Rubbifh, in Fields and cultivated Grounds — very
common. June to September. A.

SONCHUS lævis minor paucioribus laciniis.
R. S. 163.
SONCHUS *oleraceus.* H. F 294. β.
Smooth Sow-thiftle with lefs jagged Leaves.
On Rubbifh, in Fields and cultivated Grounds ——
June to September. A.

L　　　　SONCHUS

SONCHUS repens, multis Hieracium majus
    R. S. 163.
    SONCHUS *arvenfis*. H. F. 295.
    Tree Sow-thiftle.
In Fields and Hedges — *common*. Auguft. P.

SORBUS fylveftris foliis domefticæ fimilis.
    R. S. 452.
    SORBUS *aucuparia*. H. F. 189.
    Mountain Afh, Quicken Tree, Roan Tree.
In the Blean Woods — *not uncommon*. May. S.

SPARGANIUM non ramofum. R. S. 437.
    SPARGANIUM *erectum*. H. F. 346. β
    Bur-reed not branched.
In the Ditches of Ham *and* Graveney Marfhes —
    common. July. P.

SPARGANIUM ramofum. R. S. 437.
    SPARGANIUM *erectum*. H. F. 346.
    Great branched Bur-reed.
In Ponds near Ewell — *not uncommon*. July. P.

SPERGULA maritima flore parvo cæruleo, femine
    vario. R. S. 351.
    ARENARIA *marina*. H. F. 169. γ.
    Small flowered Sea-fpurrey.
In Shepey Ifland — *not uncommon*. July. P.

SPER-

SPERGULA purpurea. R. S. 163.
ARENARIA *rubra*. H. F. 169.
Purple Spurrey, Purple flowered Chickweed.
On fandy Grounds in Hernhill —— *not uncommon.*
July. A.

SPHONDYLIUM. R. S. 205.
HERACLEUM *Sphondylium*. H. F. 102.
Cow Parfnep.
On the fides of Fields, and in Hedges —— common.
July. B.

STATICE montana minor. R. S. 203.
STATICE *Armeria*. H. F. 114.
Thrift, or Sea Gilly-Flower.
In all the Salt Marfhes—*very common.* July. P.

STELLARIA. R. S. 289.
CALLITRICHE *verna*. H. F. 2.
Vernal Star wort, Water wort, Star-headed Chickweed.
In the Powder Mill Streams—*common.* April. A.

STELLARIA aquatica foliis longis tenuiffimis.
R. S. 290.
CALLITRICHE *autumnalis*. H F. 2.
Autumnal Star-wort.
In the River oppofite the Gunpowder Stove —— *not uncommon.* September. A.

STRA-

STRATIOTES foliis Afari, femine rotundo.
R. S. 290.
HYDROCHARIS *Morfus ranæ*. H F. 372.
Frog-bit.
In the Dykes of Ham *and* Graveney Marfhes ——
common. June. P.

SYMPHYTUM magnum. R. S. 230.
SYMPHYTUM *officinale*. H. F. 68.
Comfiey.
On the Banks of the Powder Mill Waters—*uncommon.*
July. P.

T.

TAMNUS racemofa, flore minore luteo palle-
fcente. R. S. 261.
TAMUS *communis*. H. F. 369.
Black Briony.
Under Hedges, and among Bufhes—common. June. P.

TANACETUM. R. S. 188.
TANACETUM *vulgare*. H. F. 310.
Common Tanfy.
By Way fides, near Queen Court *and* Uplees — *very
uncommon.* Auguft. P.

TAXUS. R. S. 445.
TAXUS *baccata*. H. F. 372.
' The Yew Tree.
In Woods and Hedges on a chalky Soil —— *common.*
April. S. THA-

THALICTRUM feu Thalietrum majus. R. S.
203.
THALICTRUM *flavum.* H. F. 216.
Meadow Rue.
In the fhooting Meadow Stream —— *uncommon.*
June. P.

TITHYMALUS characias Amygdaloides. R. S..
312.
EUPHORBIA *Amygdaloides.* H. F. 184.
Wood Spurge.
In Woods, and under Hedges in Ofpringe —— *very*
common. April. P.

TITHYMALUS heliofcopius. R. S. 313.
EUPHORBIA *Heliofcopia.* H. F. 183.
Sun Spunge, or Wart-wort.
In Meadows, and on Dunghills — common. July. A.

TITHYMALUS-leptophyllos. R. S. 313.
EUPHORBIA *exigua.* H. F. 182.
Dwarf Spurge, Small annual Spurge.
In Corn fields and Gardens —— common. July. A.

TITHYMALUS parvus annuus, foliis fubrotundis,
non crenatis, Peplus dictus. R. S. 313.
EUPHORBIA *Peplus.* H. F. 182.
Petty Spurge.
In cultivated Grounds —— common. July. A.

L 3   TITHY.

TITHYMALUS platyphyllos Fuchsii. R. S.
312.
EUPHORBIA *platyphyllos*. H. F. 184.
Broad leaved Spurge.
In Corn fields near Thorn Creek —— *common.*
July. P

TORMENTILLA. R. S. 257.
TORMENTILLA *erecta*. H. F. 197.
Tormentil Septfoil.
In Woods and Hedges — *common.* June. P.

TORMENTILLA reptans. R. S. 257.
- TORMENTILLA *reptans*. H. F. 198.
Creeping Tormentil.
In Broom fields at Hernhill — *common.* July. P.

TRAGOPOGON luteum. R. S. 171.
TRAGOPOGON *pratense*. H. F. 293.
Yellow Goat's Beard, Go to Bed at Noon.
In Fields and Pastures — *common.* June. B.

TRAGOPOGON purpureum. R S. 172.
TRAGOPOGON *porrifolium*. H. F. 293.
Purple Goat's Beard.
In a Marsh near Sheernefs —— *uncommon.*
June. B.

TRICHO-

TRICHOMANES. R. S. 119.

ASPLENIUM *Trichomanes.* H. F. 385.

Englifh black Maiden-Hair.

On the Walls of the Church *and* Abby——*not common.* P.

TRIFOLIUM arvenfe humile fpicatum feu. Lagopus. R. S. 330.

TRIFOLIUM *arvenfe.* H. F. 285.

Hare's Foot, or Hare's Foot Trefoil.

Upon Beacon Hill — *not uncommon.* July. A.

TRIFOLIUM cochleatum folio cordato maculato. R. S. 333.

MEDICAGO *arabica.* H. F. 288.

Heart Trefoil, or Clover.

In the Abby Meadows—*not uncommon.* June. A.

TRIFOLIUM cochleatum modiolis fpinofis. R. S. 333.

MEDICAGO *arabica.* H. F. 288. γ.

Hedge-hog Trefoil, or Clover.

In Paftures near Sheernefs—*not common.* May. A.

TRIFOLIUM fragiferum. R. S. 329.

TRIFOLIUM *fragiferum.* H. F. 286.

Strawberry Trefoil.

In the Abby Meadows — *common.* Auguft. P.

TRIFO-

TRIFOLIUM floſculis albis, in glomerulis ob-
longis aſperis, cauliculis próxime adnatis.
R S. 329
TRIFOLIUM ſcabrum. H. F. 285.
Oval headed Trefoil.

In Paſtures in Shepey — *common* June. A.

TRIFOLIUM lupulinum alterum minus. R. S.
330.
TRIFOLIUM *procumbens.* H. F. 287.
The leſſer Hop Trefoil, Decumbent Trefoil.

In Meadows — common. May to Auguſt. P.

TRIFOLIUM lupulinum minimum. R. S. 331.
TRIFOLIUM *filiforme.* H F 287.
Small Trefoil.

On gravelly Banks beyond South Street — *uncommon.*
May A.

TRIFOLIUM pratenſe album R. S. 327.
TRIFOLIUM *repens.* H. F. 283.
Dutch Clover, White flowered Meadow Trefoil.

In Fields and Meadows —— *very common.* May to
. September P

TRIFOLIUM pratenſe luteum capitulo Lupuli, vel
agrarium. R. S. 330.
TRIFOLIUM *agrarium.* H. F. 286.
. Hop Trefoil,

On Beacon Hill — *not uncommon.* June. A.

TRIFO-

TRIFOLIUM pratenfe purpureum. R. S. 328.
 TRIFOLIUM *pratenfe*. H. F. 284.
Common Purple or Honey-fuckle Trefoil.
In Fields and Meadows——very common. May to
 September. P.

TRIFOLIUM purpureum majus, folis longioribus
 et anguftioribus, floribus faturatioribus.
 R. S. 328.
 TRIFOLIUM *medium*. H. F. 284.
Long leaved Purple Trefoil with deeper coloured
 Flowers.
In Byfing Wood, *and by Field fides in* Ofpringe ——
 not uncommon. July. P.

TRIFOLIUM ftellatum glabrum. R. S. 329.
 TRIFOLIUM *maritimum*. H. F. 284.
Teafel-headed Trefoil.
On Shellnefs *in* Shepy — *uncommon.* June. P.

TURRITIS muralis minor. R. S. 294.
 TURRITIS *hirfuta*. H. F. 254.
Hairy Tower Muftard.
On old Walls at Colkins *in* Boughton—*very uncom-
 mon.* May. B.

TUSSILAGO. R. S. 173.
 TUSSILAGO *Farfara*. H. F. 315.
Common Colt's Foot.
In moift Fields — very common. April. P.
          TYPHA.

TYPHA. RS. 436.
  TYPHA *latifolia.* H. F. 345.
  Great Cat's Tail, or Reed Mace.
On the sides of Ponds, and in Dykes — very common.
  July. P.

TYPHA paluftris media. R. S. 436.
  TYPHA *anguftifolia.* H. F. 345.
  Narrow leaved Cat's Tail.
In the Ditches at Ewell *and* Nagden—*not uncommon.*
  July. P.

V.

VALERIANA fylveftris major. R. S. 200.
  VALERIANA *officinalis.* H. F. 12.
  Great wild Valerian.
On the Banks of Ofpringe River — *not uncommon.*
  June. P.

VALERIANA fylveftris minor. R. S. 200.
  VALERIANA *dioica* H. F. 12.
  Small wild or Marfh Valerian.
On the Banks of the fhooting Meadow Stream——
  common. June. P.

VALERIANELLA arvenfis præcox humilis
  femine compreffo, five Lactuca agnina.
  R. S 201.
  VALERIANA *Locufta* H. F. 12.
  Lamb's Lettuce, or Corn Sallad.
In Corn fields, and rich cultivated Ground — common.
  May. A.   VALE-

VALERIANELLÆ vulgaris fpecies major, ferotina. R. S. 201.
  VALERIANA *Locufta.* H. F. 13. β.
Late flowering Lambs Lettuce, or Corn Sallad.
In the Corn fields between Ore *and* Harty-ferry—*not common.* July. A.

VERBASCUM flore albo parvo. R. S. 287.
  VERBASCUM *Lychnitis.* H. F. 76.
Hoary Mullein, or white Mullein.
On old Walls at Davington—*not common.* July. B.

VERBASCUM mas latifolium luteum. R.S. 287.
  VERBASCUM *Thapfus.* H. F. 75.
Great white Mullein, High Taper, Cows Lungwort.
On dry Banks by Road fides — *common.* July. B.

VERBASCUM nigrum flore parvo, apicibus purpureis. R. S. 288.
  VERBASCUM *nigrum.* H. F. 76.
Sage-leaved black Mullein.
On the fides of Chalk fields in Ofpringe — *very uncommon. As you afcend St.* Martin's-Hill *near* Canterbury — *plentifully.* July. P.

VERBENA vulgaris. R. S. 236.
  VERBENA *officinalis.* H. F. 505.
Vervain.
By Road fides and Foot paths—very common. July. P.

VERBESINA feu Cannabina aquatica flore minus
    pulchro elatior. R. S. 187.
  BIDENS *tripartita*. H. F. 309.
  Trifid Water-hemp Agrimony.
In marfhy watery Places — common. July. A.

VERBESINA pulchriore flore luteo. R. S. 187.
  BIDENS *cernua*. H. F. 309.
  Whole leaved Water-hemp Agrimony.
In Dykes near the Town Key—*common.* Auguft. A.

VERONICA aquatica anguftifolia minor. R. S.
    280.
  VERONICA *fcutellata*. H. F. 5.
  Narrow leaved Water Speedwell, or Brooklime.
In wet Ditches and marfhy Ground—common. June. P.

VERONICA aquatica longifolia media. R.S. 280.
  VERONICA *Anagallis*. H. F. 5.
  The middle long leaved Water Speedwell, or
    Brooklime.
In the Abby *Ditches — common.* July. P.

VERONICA aquatica rotundifolia Becabunga
    dicta minor. R. S. 280.
  VERONICA *Becabunga*. H F. 4.
  Common Brooklime.
In wet Ditches and fmall running Waters ——— very
    common. May. P.

VERONICA

VERONICA Chamædrys fylveftris dicta. R.S. 281.
VERONICA *Chamædrys.* H. F. 5.
Wild Germander.
In Fields and Meadows — very common. May. P.

VERONICA floribus fingularibus, in oblongis
pediculis, Chamædryfolia. R S 279.
VERONICA *agreftis.* H. F. 6.
Germander Speedwell, or Chickweed.
*In Fields, on Rubbifh, and in cultivated Ground ——
common,* May. A.

VERONICA flofculis fingularibus Hederulæ folio,
Morfus gallinæ minor dicta. R. S. 280.
VERONICA *hederifolia.* H. F. 6.
Ivy leaved Speedwell, or fmall Henbit.
In dry Fields, and on old Walls—common. April. A.

VERONICA mas fupina et vulgatiffima. R. S.
281.
VERONICA *officinalis.* H. F. 4.
The Male Speedwell, or Fluellin.
In barren dry Fields — common. May. P.

VERONICA pretenfis minor ; five Betonica Pauli.
R. S. 279.
VERONICA *ferpyllifolia.* H. F. 4.
Little, or fmooth Speedwell, or Paul's Betony.
In Fields and Meadows — common. May. P.

M   VIBUR-

VIBURNUM. R. S. 460
  VIBURNUM *Lantana.* **H. F.** 112.
  The pliant Mealy, or Way-faring Tree.
In Hedges — common. May. S.

VICIA. R S. 320.
  VICIA *fativa.* **H F.** 278.
  Common Vetch, or Tare.
In Fields among Corn — not uncommon. June. A.

VICIA fepium perennis. **R. S.** 320.
  VICIA *fepium.* **H. F** 278.
  Bufh Vetch.
In bufhy Places and Hedges — common. May. P.

VICIA minima præcox Parifienfium. **R. S.** 321.
  FRVUM *folomenfe.* **H. F.** 279.
  Spring Tare.
In Ofpringe *Chalk Pits — common.* April. P.

VICIA fylveftris five Cracca major. **R. S.** 321.
  VICIA *lathyroides.* **H F.** 279.
  Strangle Tare, or Wild Vetch.
In fandy Fields in Hernhill —— *not uncommon.*
  May. A.

VINCA

VINCA Pervinca minor. R. S. 268.
VINCA *minor*. H. F. 77.
Periwinkle.

In Cades *Wood, and Hedges in* Preston *and* Ospringe
— *common* April. P. With a white Flower,
near the 39th Mile Stone — *very uncommon.*

VIOLA bicolor arvensis. R. S. 366.
VIOLA *tricolor*. H. F 331. β
Pansies, Heart's-ease, Two Faces under a Hood.
In sandy Corn fie'ds at Hernhill —— *common.* August. A.

VIOLA martia inodora sylvestris. R. S. 364.
VIOLA *canina*. H. F. 331.
Wild or Dogs Violet.
In Woods and under Hedges—very common. April. P.

VIOLA martia hirsuta inodora. R. S. 365.
VIOLA *hirta*. H. F. 330.
Hairy Violet.
In the new Wood at Cades *in* Ospringe — *plen tfully.*
March. P.

VIOLA martia alba. R. S. 364.
VIOLA *odorata*. H. F. 330. β.
White Violet.
*Under dry Hedges and Banks, by Way sides — not un-
common,* March. P

VIOLA

VIOLA martia purpurea. R. S. 364.
 VIOLA *odorata*. H. F. 330.
 Purple fweet Violet.
Under Hedges, and in Fields —— *very common.*
 March. P.

VIOLA tricolor. R. S. 361.
 VIOLA *tricolor*. H. F. 331.
 Panfies, Three Faces under a Hood.
In Corn fields at Ore, *and in Gardens* —— *common.*
 June. A.

VIRGA aurea. R. S. 176.
 SOLIDAGO *Virga aurea*. H. F. 318.
 Common Golden Rod.
In Woods and Hedges — *common.* Auguft. P.

VISCUM. R. S. 464.
 VISCUM *album*. H. F. 367.
 Miffel, or Miffeltoe.
On Trees, efpecially in Orchards —— *common.*
 May. S.

VULNERARIA ruftica. R. S. 325.
 ANTHYLLIS *Vulneraria* H. F. 273.
 Kidney Vetch, or Ladies Finger.
About Byfing Wood —— *common.* July. P.

ULMA

U.

ULMARIA. R. S. 259.

SPIRÆA *Ulmaria.* H. F. 191.

Meadow fweet.

In moift Meadows in Davington—*common.* July. P.

ULMUS folio glabro.

ULMUS *glabra.* H. F. 95. β.

The fmooth leaved or Wych Elm.

In Hedges— not uncommon. April. S.

ULMUS folio latiffimo fcabro. R. S. 469.

ULMUS *glabra.* H. F. 95.

The Wych Hazel, or broad-leaved Elm.

In Hedges at Throwleigh—*uncommon.* April. S.

ULMUS vulgatiffima, folio lato fcabro. R. S. 468.

ULMUS *campeftris.* H. F. 94.

The common Elm.

In Hedges —— *very common.* April. S.

URTICA minor. R. S. 140.

URTICA *urens.* H. F. 355.

The leffer Stinging Nettle.

In cultivated and uncultivated Ground — very common.

Auguft. A.

M 3 URTICA

URTICA racemifera major perennis. R. S. 139.
URTICA *dioica*. H. F. 355.
The common Stinging Nettle.
-*Under Hedges, and on Rubbish* —— *very common*
July. P.

PLANTS OMITTED.

* CALENDULA *officinalis*. Lin. Syft. Nat II.
p. 577.
Garden Marigold.
On the Beach at St. Margaret's *at* Cliff; *plentifully*
And in a Field at Woodnefborow—*very*
uncommon. June. A.

CRAMBE maritima braffica folio. R. S. 307.
CRAMBE *maritima*. H. F. 260.
Sea Colewort.
At St Margaret's *at* Cliff—*uncommon.* June. P.

HYDROCERATOPHYLLON folio afpero qua-
tuor cornibus armato R. S. 135.
CERATOPHYLLUM *demerfum*. H. F. 357.
Horned Pond-weed.
In Marfh Dykes —— *Common.* June. P.

* MYAGRUM. R. S 302.
MYAGRUM *fativum*. H. F. 242.
Gold of Pleafure.
Near Sandwich, *among the Flax* —— *plentifully.*
June. A. TRI-

TRIFOLLIUM luteum lupulinum. R. S. 331.
  MEDICAGO *lupulina.* H. F. 288.
  Melilot Trefoil.
In Paths near Weftwood — *not common.* May to
  Auguft. A.

CAUCULIS nodofa echinato femine. R. S. 220.
  TORDILIUM *nodofum.* H. F. 98.
  Knotted Parfley.
By the Road fide at Minfter *in* Shepey—*not common*
  May. A.

LINARIA antirrhinum dicta. R. S. 283.
  ANTIRRHINUM *minus.* H. F. 238.
  The leaft Toad Flax.
In a Corn field near Whitehill, Selling —— *uncom-
  mon.* A.

SENECIO minor latiore folio, five montana.
  R. S. 178.
  SENECIO *fylvaticus.* H. F. 316.
  Mountain Groundfel.
In Badgen Wood—*not common.* Auguft. A.

OENANTHE aquatica triflora. R. S 220.
  OENANTHE *fiftulofa.* H. F. 104. β.
  The leffer Water Dropwort.
In Ditches at Graveney — *common.* July. P.

FOSSILIA SHEPEIANA.

A

SHORT VIEW

OF THE

FOSSIL BODIES

Native and Extraneous,

OF THE

ISLAND

OF

SHEPEY,

IN THE

COUNTY OF KENT.

Quicquid sub terra est in apricum proferet ætas.

INTRODUCTION.

*T*H E *Iſland of* Shepey, *with the annexed Penin-*
ſulas of Harty *and* Elmly, *ſurrounded by the*
Waters of the Thames, *the* Medway, *and the* Sea, *is*
upwards of Thirty Miles in Circumference, about
Thirteeen in Length from Shellneſs *to* Sheerneſs, *and*
in its greateſt Breadth about Six. It bath long been
noted for producing large Quantities of Sheep (from whence
probably it derived its Name) as well as Corn; and
exhibits to the inquiſitive Naturaliſt a moſt deſirable
Spot, by affording on its Surface many rare Plants,
and more eſpecially in the Bowels of its Northern
Cliffs, *ſo great a Quantity and Variety of* Foſſils, *both*
native and extraneous, as are ſcarcely to be paralled.

Theſe Cliffs are in Length about Six Miles from Eaſt
to Weſt, gradually declining at each End; the more
elevated Parts whereof reach about two-thirds of their
extenſion, and are, at the very higheſt of them about
Minſter, *not leſs than Thirty Yards in perpendicular*
Height above the Beach or Shore, and being compoſed
of Clay, and conſtantly waſhed at their Baſis by the
Tides

Tides which beat against them more especially when driven by strong Easterly Winds, they are continually wasting more or less, and falling down upon the Shore, where the Clay being by degrees washed away, the Fossils are left in great Abundance. So great is the Loss of the Land at the highest Parts, that sometimes near an Acre of it hath sunk down at once, though these Falls are indeed extraordinary.

Minster, Shurland, *and* Warden, *are the three Manors to which these Cliffs appertain, the Proprietors whereof hire them out to different Owners of Coperas Works, who employ the neighbouring Poor to collect the* Pyrites *or* Copperas Stone *upon the Beach, at the Rate of about a Shilling per Bushel, which they deposit in Heaps, when collected, until a Quantity sufficient to load a Hoy is procured, when it is measured and paid for.*

These Coperas Gatherers, from the Author's first Visits were induced to preserve and carry home every Thing that seemed to their Apprehension somewhat particular, and having since met with Encouragement, and acquired some Information relative to what was most desirable by the Curious, they have generally from that Time reserved such, until Inquiries have been made for them. Many rare Specimens, both native and extraneous, far beyond any equal Space of Ground,

perhaps

perhaps the Universe can produce, are by these means preserved. Indeed, more may thus be obtained, at a very easy Expence, than by the most diligent Fossilists alone, as they cannot allow due Time to examine the Shore sufficiently. This is evidently confirmed by comparing the Specimens from this Coast, recited in the Works of our most celebrated * Naturalists, with those in the ensuing Catalogue. The Author doubts not that many curious Specimens have escaped his Inquiries, and as the Cliffs are daily dropping their Contents more or less, he is fully assured that there will always remain a Variety sufficient to gratify every Lover of the Study, whenever they may choose to take a Trip thither. But alas! One disagreeable Circumstance attending a considerable Part of the Fossils here collected, is, that they are so much impregnated with Pyritical Matter, that after being for some Time placed in a Cabinet, the Salts thereof shoot and entirely destroy them. Happy would it be, could some certain Remedy be discovered whereby this Accident might be prevented. The Loss of many valuable Specimens by this Cause, together with his Distance from any inquisitive and able Naturalists, at last induced the Author to dispose of his whole Collection to INGHAM FOSTER, *Esq;*

---

* Dr. Grew, Mr. Llhuyd, Mr. Petiver, Dr. Woodward, Mr. Dale, and Dr. Hill.

Merchant

Merchant of London, *where it now forms no incon-*
fiderable Part of that Gentleman's very valuable
Cabinet.

He, many Years fince, entertained Thoughts of
publifhing a defcriptive Catalogue of all the Foffils
there, by him collected, but was prevented, as well by
more neceffary Attachments as the Difficulty of the
Undertaking: However, it having been intimated to
him that a concife Account of them wou'd not be
deemed an unacceptable Appendix to his PLANTÆ
FAVERSHAMIENSES, *in which feveral of the*
Shepey *Plants are recited, as no fpecial Account of*
thefe Foffils hath been offered to the Public, and as
thofe that have been already noted by the before cited
Authors are difperfed in their Works, and as many
others have not as yet been publifhed, he complied with
the Propofal, and fet about revifing his Notes and
Obfervations, and now offers thi fhort Account of the
Difcoveries made there in his annual Vifits for above
thefe Thirty Years paft; at firft folely for the Purpofe
of collecting thefe elegant Bodies, and afterwards to
fuperintend his private Affairs, having acquired fome
Property in the Ifland, not far diftant from the Cliffs.

What the candid Reader may expect in the following
Catalogue is, a general Account of the Variety of the
Foffil Bodies, *both native and extraneous, reduced into*

N   *fome*

some Order under particular Heads, with Notice of their degrees of Rarity. If what is offered shall afford any Information worthy the attention of the Lovers of Natural History, the Author will think himself sufficiently rewarded for this Attempt of exhibiting the Out-lines of a Work which merits the Abilities of a Person of more Judgment and greater Leisure, to enlarge and perfect, than he pretends to be possessed of. He cannot conclude however, without observing, that from the contemplation of so great a Variety of extraneous Fossils discovered in these Cliffs, which were evidently the produce of very different Climates, he thinks himself rationally induced to believe, that nothing short of an universal Deluge could be a Cause adequate to such an Effect.

E. J.

FOSSILIA SHEPEIANA.

NATIVE FOSSILS.

The CLIFFS.

THESE are compofed of three different Strata of brown Clay; the uppermoft is of the lighteft Colour, and moft friable; the loweft darkeft, and of a clofer Texture.

PYRITÆ.

Coperas Stones, are the moft frequent of all t (Foffils of the Cliffs: They are of various Forms and Sizes; round, botryoide, flat, varying in every L gree, as well in Figure as Colour, and impregnating moft of the other Foffils found here.

LUDUS HELMONTII:

The Waxen Vein ; Nodules of which are lodged in the Cliffs in great Numbers; they are generally flat and oval, and of various Sizes, fometimes exceed-ing two Feet in length, all are covered with Coats

N 2

in

in the Cliffs, but are frequently feen denudated on the Beach, the *Tali* are of different Sizes and Forms, generally they pafs ftrait from one flat Surface of the Nodule to the other; in fome there is a double Set of them, running only half through the Body, with intermediate fparry Partitions, which being generally of a waxen Colour, at firft gave this Nodule its Name. The Number of the *Tali* in different Nodules are indeterminate; both the *Tali* and *Septa* vary in Colour in different Specimens — they are very common.

BEZOAR MINERALE.

Bodies, which are cruftated, ferrugineous, and of a rounded Form, covered with various Crufts of the Colour of the Clay of the Cliffs, and of different Sizes — Thefe are common.

CALCULI.

Pebbles. Amongft the numbers on the Beach, there have been fome Specimens collected, which by polifhing have proved very elegant.

SELENITES.

Selenite, is found here in great Plenty, chiefly of the columnar fort, fome Specimens exceed fix Inches in length, but moft are of fhorter dimen-
fions,

fions, which are common. The rhomboidal Sort
is not near fo common.

LEPASTRUM. D. HILL.

The Starry Waxen Vein, is a Foffil peculiar to
thefe Cliffs, not having as yet been difcovered elfe-
where to the Author's Knowledge. Dr. *Hill* hath
made from their Forms three Sorts of it, to which
others might be added if nicely attended to. It is
ever affixed to the Septa of the Ludus Helmontii,
where the Fiffures are fo far divided as to permit
the Stars to fhoot. The largeft Specimens do not
exceed three Inches in Length, and thefe are very
rare; thofe are generally of a much lefs Size that
are common.

SUCCINUM.

Amber, is very uncommon; a few Specimens
only, and thofe fmall and tranfparent, are to be
found here.

EXTRANEOUS FOSSILS.

VEGETABLES.

LIGNUM FOSSILE.

Foffil Wood, in large Maffes, feemingly of Oak
from its Grain, even to above three Feet in Length,

is plentifully difperfed on the Beach, and generally impregnated with pyritical Matter.

EQUISETUM.

Horfe-tail, Joints of the naked Species, are fometimes found even to the Length of three Inches, but they are uncommon.

FRUCTUS VARII.

Foffil Fruits, of very different Kinds, are here collected, in Variety and Number exceeding all that have been mentioned by Writers on this Branch of Natural Hiftory: Many of them have been drawn and compared with recent ones, in a particular Account given of them by the Author's late learned Friend, Dr. *James Parfons*, in the Philofophical Tranfactions — Vol. L Part I. p 396. Thefe have by fome been imagined mere Sports of Nature amongft the Coperas; but as all the Specimens have not the misfortune to be impregnated by it, fome few, and thofe very elegant ones, being entirely free from it, and petrified, that Conceit without further Difcuffion, muft fall to the Ground.

ARISTÆ.

Ears of Corn, fome fmall Species, are fometimes to be met with, imperfect and impregnated with the Pyrites, but they are not common.

MYCE-

MYCETITÆ.

The Mushroom Stone. Here are two Kinds, the Conoide and Difcoide, both fmall, and the firft is by far the moft frequently to be found.

ANIMALIUM PARTES.

ELEPHAS.

The Elephant. A confiderable Number of the Bones of this very laige Animal have been difco-vered on the Eaftern Shore, a Mile from the Cliffs, on the ∽uthor's Manor of *Nutts,* in *Laysdown*, an Account of which may be feen in the Philofophical Tianfactions — Vol. xlviii. part ii. page 626.

TESTUDO.

The Tortoife. Two varieties have been found under the Cliffs, one of a more convexed Form, the other more depreffed ; both are extreamly rare.

PISCIUM PARTES.

The Heads of Fifh, from a very fmall Size to that of a middling Cod, are not unfrequent.

Palates of Fifh, fome oval, others of a fquarifh form, when perfect, or nearly fo, are very uncommon ;

common; but fmall Portions of them, efpecially of the fquare Sort are common: To thefe laft, Mr. *Llhuyd* hath given the whimfical Name of *Scopula littoralis*, and to thofe of the firft kind, *Bufonitæ*. In the Gentleman's Magazine for May, 1755, p. 409, is a Plate exhibiting both Kinds, in fine Prefervation.

Teeth of Fifh, ufually called *Sharks Teeth*, are plentifully met with, except thofe of a large Size, which are very uncommon.

Back Bones of Fifh, are very common in feparate Joints, but with three or more united, are uncommon.

Parts of the Bodies of Fifh, with the Scales on them, are not very uncommon, but none entire have come to the Author's Knowledge.

Tails of Fifh, are frequently collected, and fome few with a Vertebra united to them; there are very few of a large Size.

CANCRI MACROURI.

Lobfters, are not uncommon, but none of the Specimens are perfect; the Bodies and Tails united are not fo frequent as when feparated; the Claws are alfo found feparately of various Sizes, but generally much injured.

Prawns

Prawns, are very rare; they are nearly perfect, and confiderably larger than thofe taken recent on the oppofite Coaft of the Ifle of *Thanet*.

CANCRI BRACHYURI.

Foffil Crabs. Before the Publication of Dr. *Hill's* Hiftory of *Foffils*, thefe were extreamly rare in England, but fince that Time, thoufands of Specimens here collected, have paffed through the Author's Hands. There are two or three Varieties, but all common except very fair Specimens, which are ftill very rare; their Size varies from that of a fmall Bean, to that of the common *Crab* of the Coaft; fome of them, efpecially the fmaller ones, are impregnated by the *Pyrites*.

ECHINITÆ.

Echinites, here are the *Ovarius*, *Galeatus*, *Pileatus*, *Cordatus*, and *Placentiformis*; but all of them are very rare, efpecially the laft.

The Spines, are of the foliated Kind, and that Sort named by Mr. *Lhuyd*, *Volvola*—both are rare.

ASTERIAS.

The Star Fifh of five Rays, has not yet been found entire, and its fingle Rays are uncommon.

ASTROITÆ

ASTROITÆ ET ASTEROPODIUM.

Star Stones, with depreſſed Rays, and the Roots of them are very uncommon; the Specimens of the latter Kind were ſo imperfect, that without better Information the Author was at a Loſs how to place them in his Collection.

BELEMNITES.

Belemnite, only one Specimen, and that imperfect, hath hitherto been diſcovered.

CONCHYLIA.

TUBULI MARINI.

Worm Shells, of various contorted Forms, generally of a ſmall Size, ſome with their Shells, others denudated, frequently impregnated with the Coperas, are common.

LAPIS SYRINGOIDES.

The piped Waxen Vein, externally appears like the *Ludus Helmontii,* being found in incruſted Nudoles; they are evidently Oak that had firſt been eroded by Sea Worms, and afterwards their Perforations filled with Pyritical Matter and *Spar,*

ſimilar

fimilar to the *Waxen Vein*, furrounding each Per-
foration; thefe are very common.

CONCHYLIA UNIVALVIA.

DENTALIA.

The Tooth Shells, generally fmall, about an Inch
long, curving towards the Apex in the more perfect Specimens, fome covered with their Shells,
and others denudated, both Sorts are common.

PATELLA.

The Limpet, is a very rare Foffil, having only
once been collected; the Specimen was fmall, of
the ftriated Sort, and fomewhat imperfect.

NAUTILUS.

The chambered Nautilus, is a common Foffil of
thefe Cliffs. Thefe vary in Size from that of Hazel-
Nut to that of a Man's Head, moft commonly
they have their pearly Shell, and are often im-
merfed in Nodules; there are alfo fome fmall ones
found of a ferrugineous Colour; very few of the
large ones are perfect, having received Injury by
compreffion.

ORTHO-

ORTHOCERATITES.

Small Fragments feemingly of this *Genus* are found here, but very uncommon, the Chambers or Partitions appear to be united by a Dove tail Suture.

TUBULI CONCAMERATI.

Cylindrical Bodies, with feveral Concamerations paffing tranfverfly through them, are generally of the Size of a Swan's Quill, and about two or three Inches in Length, fome petrified, others wholly pyritical, and are not uncommon.

COCHLEÆ.

Snail Shells, with a fhort as well as with a produced Clavicle, fome with their Shells, others denudated, are generally of a fmall Size, and impregnated by the *Pyrites*, and are uncommon.

TROCHI

The Topfhells, are of different Forms, fome flatter, others more elevated, of various Sizes, fome with Shells on, others denudated, moft are impregnated with *Pyrites*, and are common.

CONCHA

CONCHA VENERIS.

The Cowry. This is fmall, denudated, pyritical, and extremely rare.

BUCCINA.

Whilkes, are found in confiderable Quantities, varying in Form and Size, but generally fmall.
The Opercula are fometimes, though rarely feen.

NERITÆ.

The Nerites, are common; and generally impregnated with Pyrites.

TURBINES.

The Screw Shells, and cafts of them without the Shell, of various Sizes, and moftly impregnated with Pyrites, are very common.

CONCHYLIA BIVALVIA.

OSTREA.

Foffil Oyfters; generally of a fmall Size, are found here, but very uncommon; although the whole Coaft is covered with recent ones.

O   CONCHÆ

CONCHÆ ANOMIÆ.

These Shells in great variety, tho' generally of a small Size, and impregnated with the Pyrites, are very common.

PECTUNCULI.

Cockles, smooth, striated, and fasciated, of a small Size, are found in tolerable Plenty; but fair and large Specimens are uncommon.

TELLINÆ.

The Wedge Shell. Small Specimens of which, generally denudated and pyritical, are very common.

MUSCULI.

Muscles. These are extreamly rare, a few large Specimens, and one only of the common Muscle have been hitherto met with; although the Coast abounds with the latter.

PINNÆ.

The Sea Wing. Only small Fragments of this Shell have as yet been discovered, and these are very rare.

F I N I S.

INDEX

OF THE

ENGLISH NAMES.

A.

Arsmart,

C.

Can-

Cow-

Figwort,

G.

Glafs.

Hep-b

Ivy,

b 2

b 3   Nettle-

Orchis,

S.

Sea

Sow-

Tormentil

Venus-

Wood

INDEX

OF THE

LINNÆAN NAMES.

A.

Anethum

INDEX.

Calen-

C.

Cheiran-

d

Cratægus

Equi-

Frankenia

I.

L.

Linum

Meliffa

Onopor-

Pedicu-

Poten-

e   Scleran-

Sonchus

T.

Trifolium

Veronica

ERRATA.

The candid Reader is defired to correct thefe Errors and Omiffions.

Page line
4   20 *after* marina *add* β.
17   9 *for* Pluckley *read* Hedcorne
28   19 *after* Sandwich *add* and on Shellnefs.
36   4 *after* Sittingbourn *add* and on the Standard Key.
42   25 *after* Deal *add* and on Shellnefs
49   20 *for* eleganiffimum *read* elegantiffimum.
—   22 *for* montenum *read* montanum.
56   22 *after* 304 *add* γ.
57   2 *after* 304 *add* δ
59   5 *for* *uncommon* read *common.*
—   12 *for* *common* read *uncommon.*
73   4 *for* Fairbrook *read* Luddenham
76   21 *after* *plentifully* add *on* Badgen Downs, *sparingly.*
88   14 *for* granineum *read* gramineum.
144 16 *for* *uncommon* read *common.*

Omitted to be inferted in their proper Places.

ANTIRRHINUM anguftifolium fylveftre.
   R. S. * 283.
   ANTIRRHINUM *Orontium.*   H. F. 239.
The leaft Snapdragon, or Calf's-fnout.
In a Corn field at Luddenham — *uncommon.*
   July. A.

CASSIDA paluftris vulgatior flore cæruleo.
-   R. S. 244.
   SCUTELLARIA *galericulata.* H. F. 231.
Hooded Willow-herb.
In a moift Hedge at Chartham Hatch—*uncommon.*
   Auguft. P.

Ingram Content Group UK Ltd.
Milton Keynes UK
UKHW022011160523
421870UK00005B/46